To Evie

I'll never forget your daddy
and the love we shared, but you are my future ...

Make your own way, my darling daughter.

Love Mummy xxx

March 2007

The first time I saw Paul Hunter, he was 18 and I was 21. I needed a lift into town for a night out, and a friend said, 'My little cousin will drive us in.' I got into his blue sports car and my first impression was, 'He's just a kid.' His cousin said he was a snooker player, and I asked, 'As a job? That's not a real job – that's a hobby!'

The last time I saw Paul Hunter, he was 27 and I was 31. By then, he was my husband and the father of our baby daughter. We'd had the world at our feet for years, but it was slipping away fast. Paul was lying in a bed in a Huddersfield hospice, ravaged and exhausted, finally giving up his 18-month fight with cancer. I held his hand and said, 'It's time to go, darling. Just close your eyes.'

This is the story of everything that lay between those two events: the love and the laughter; the glitter and the fame; the pain and the fear; the terror and the loss. It's a story that doesn't end with death, that doesn't end because one of us is no longer here. It's a story about love ...

It wasn't love at first sight. Not for either of us. When I first met Paul Hunter he was just a daft boy. He had too much time on his hands, too little structure in his life, and too many people telling him he was God's gift. Yet he had that smile. I can see it, feel it, even now. There was a magic about him that seemed to make him shine from the inside out. It wasn't just his looks – although he was gorgeous, with floppy blond hair, sparkly green eyes and a cheeky grin. It wasn't just his success – although by the time I met him he was well on the way to fame and fortune. It was the way he charmed everyone he met, from old ladies to lads in the pub, to shopkeepers and taxi drivers. He didn't have a bad bone in his body.

I have so many beautiful memories. The best one of all is the living, breathing one I'm holding in my arms right now: Evie Rose, our baby girl. Paul and I ended up loving each other so much that there just had to be concrete proof, and I'm looking at her. As I sit here in an almost empty house getting ready to move, surrounded by packing cases and boxes, of course I grieve for all the happy times I spent here with Paul, but I won't be broken by the memories of them.

Paul knew how to live; and he packed more into his few short years on earth than most people do in a lifetime. He made people happy. He made me happy. I could sit here in tears – and goodness knows there are plenty of times I feel like it. Who wouldn't grieve for a husband torn away from them after only two years of marriage? Who wouldn't feel their heart had been ripped out after 18 months spent watching him dragged to hell and back by terminal cancer?

I think these things sitting on the floor. I realize by Evie's whimperings that I'm holding her too tightly, rocking back and forward a bit too frantically. She'll never know her daddy, and he'll never know what she grows up to be, but I won't condemn her to life with a mother who only lives in the past.

I'm going to take the devotion that Paul gave me and shower our daughter with it. I'm going to teach her to be strong and fill her up with so much love that she will be able to take on the world one day. I'll tell her all about her dad and make her proud to be his daughter – and she in turn will form part of his amazing, unique legacy.

Chapter One

23 March 2005

It was a beautiful early spring morning. I got up, showered, got dressed, just as I would on any other day. I shouted to my husband Paul to get up too as I went downstairs to make breakfast. He was quite quick that morning, given that he could usually sleep for England. I glanced at him as he stumbled into the kitchen, long blond hair flopping over his eyes. We'd been married almost a year, together for a lot longer, and I still got a flutter every time I looked at him – my husband!

My husband was Paul Hunter.

My husband was one of the best snooker players in the entire world.

He was famous and loved and recognized – but to me, none of that mattered when he came home at night, when the rest of the world wasn't there.

He was just the man of my dreams.

I absolutely adored him.

He came over to me behind the breakfast bar of our Leeds

1

home and grabbed a bacon sarnie off the plate, kissing me as he did it. 'Come on then,' he said. 'Let's be going, Linz.'

I pulled him towards me as he headed for the door. 'Paul,' I began, 'Whatever happens …'

He cut me off. 'It'll be fine, Linz. Everything will be fine. You've said so yourself often enough.' With that he smiled, picked up the keys to his BMW and we headed out of the door.

It took over an hour to get there, park, and make our way inside. The sign on the wall will mean lots of things to lots of different people: St James' University Hospital, commonly known to locals as Jimmy's. They might be there to have a baby, to get their broken leg fixed, to see their granny – a thousand reasons, each one so important to the person experiencing it. We didn't know what we were going to hear but, as always, I had a plan. If I prepared myself for the worst, I thought nothing could surprise me, nothing could knock me off course.

I'd already had my shock. The one that took us there. Only a couple of weeks earlier, Paul became concerned about a pain in his side. The worry was that he might be heading for a burst appendix. God, we thought, how awful would that be? But it wasn't his appendix; it was a lump. That day, in Jimmy's, one of the largest oncology centres in Europe, we were to find out whether our life could move on. There was still a bit of me that was surprised we were even in an 'oncology' centre. I wouldn't have known what the word meant until this all started. I know now. I know the definition: it's the branch of medicine that deals with tumours, including the study of their development, diagnosis, treatment and prevention.

The branch of medicine that deals with the word we all fear.

Cancer.

We walked towards the NHS waiting room and I think I was probably shaking, but it was hard to tell because Paul was shaking so much more. There was peeling paper on the walls, ancient magazines on the tables, and a coffee machine that no one was risking. The waiting room was busy. It felt old, as if no one had put any care into it for years and that made me cross. People who sit waiting there are going through a very bad time in their lives. Couldn't it have been nicer? Couldn't it have been fresh and clean and pretty? I knew I was trying to distract myself.

Paul and I were holding hands. Tightly. Sometimes I ran my hand over the top of his, back and forth. Sometimes I squeezed his fingers and smiled when he looked at me. Sometimes I gave him a little kiss on the cheek. It was all meant to comfort – but why was I trying to comfort him if everything was going to be all right?

I wanted it to be over and done with so that we could get on with our lives, be together until we were old. Another part of me didn't want to move, didn't want time to tick by. If the news was bad, I knew everything would be broken from the moment we were told.

There were people of all ages, all types, beside us. Every so often, someone nodded towards Paul, or smiled, or hesitantly said 'Hiya'. He didn't know these people and I wondered whether they recognized him as the snooker player from the telly or if there was just some sort of automatic friendship between people waiting to hear if they had cancer or not?

'You'll be fine, babes,' I said. Again.

I'd been saying it for two weeks, ever since he first got the pain in his side. I said it in the middle of the night when he woke up in a cold sweat. I said it when he came back from doing an interview in which he talked about the future. I said it to everyone else, and I said it to myself.

This was D Day. We'd staggered through the last two weeks, trying to be a normal couple, trying to forget what was going to happen that day, but we couldn't ignore it any longer. There was only one thought going through my mind: PLEASE LET EVERYTHING BE OK.

Paul walked into the consulting room and I followed. We sat down and went through the usual pleasantries, constantly aware of the folder on the doctor's desk. I tried to read things upside down, tried to read the body language of the consultant. Then the reality hit me. I actually heard what he was saying.

I had prepared myself for the worst and it happened.

Those words were being said.

Paul had cancer.

Chapter Two

March 1997

*E*ight years earlier, Paul Hunter had arrived in my world without any fanfare. It started innocently enough, but none of us know how little, everyday moments are going to join together to form the story of our lives, do we? I was working in a Leeds beauty salon at the time and probably could have won competitions as the most reliable, steady 21-year-old in the city. I'd gone to a local beauty college at 16 and worked in a salon to get experience from that point on, always taking any chance for extra responsibility, always planning ahead. I'd had a pension plan and an endowment fund since my first pay packet was put into my hand as a teenager, and I'd never taken a day off work in my life. As well as working in the salon full time during the day, I worked as an assessor and tutor in a college in the city centre at night.

One day, into this sensible, organized world flew Nicky Hunter, Paul's cousin. The door of the salon burst open and this dark-haired bundle of energy ran straight behind the reception desk and threw her arms around me. We'd met a few years earlier at college when we did some classes together but as Nicky was in the year ahead of me, we'd lost touch once she graduated. I'd always liked her, and seeing her again brought a smile to my face – she was loud, funny, and never backwards at coming forwards.

'Lindsey!' she screamed once she'd released me from a bear hug. 'Where have you been?' I hadn't been anywhere. I was in Leeds all the time but to Nicky life was only what happened around about her, so as far as she was concerned I could have been on the Moon for three years. She had known all there was to know about my life back at college, so she launched straight into the question she was most interested in.

'Are you still with Dave?' she asked. Before I got a chance to answer, she went on, 'God, that's been years now, hasn't it? I've never known anyone to have a boyfriend that long. Weren't you only about 15 when you started seeing him?'

Nicky was right. Dave had been a family friend ever since I could remember, and we'd always hung around together. About six years ago, that natural friendship turned into an equally natural relationship when he came on holiday to Spain with my friend's family. We went away as mates and came back as boyfriend and girlfriend. He was my first boyfriend. In fact, he had been my only boyfriend. And now, he was my ex-boyfriend.

'We've split up,' I told her, aware there was a queue forming behind her in the reception area.

'Don't get yourselves all worked up,' Nicky announced to the tutting customers behind her. 'I've come to book a day of beauty for my twenty-first, and I need to speak to this young lady about it *in detail.*' She shepherded me out from behind the desk and onto the sofa in the waiting area. As a junior took my place, Nicky settled down for some gossip.

'What happened, Linz?' she whispered, no doubt hoping for something juicy.

'Nothing really,' I had to admit. 'It just sort of reached an end. We weren't going anywhere, so there didn't seem much point in sticking together.'

Nicky didn't mince her words. 'Was it because he was a bit boring?'

'He wasn't boring!' I protested. 'He was just … well … normal.'

I felt I had to defend Dave; he was a genuinely nice bloke and he'd always been good to me in our years together. 'Just because he wasn't out on the town every night, clubbing and drinking, doesn't mean he was boring.'

She snorted at me. 'Ha! Maybe you've turned into him, Lindsey Fell. In fact, you were always in need of a bit of lightening up. You're a bit too serious sometimes.'

Judging by her looks and gestures, my boss was making it clear that I needed to do some work, so I got Nicky booked in for her manicure, facial and everything else she could think of, swapped phone numbers, then went back to dealing with other clients. I had a smile on my face for the rest of the day, though; Nicky had always put me in a good mood, and I was glad she was back in my life.

As soon as I got home that night, the phone rang. 'Lindsey?' said Nicky on the other end. 'I've not forgotten about you,' she said, as if it had been much more than six hours since we last spoke. 'This weekend you're coming out with me and some mates. We're going to get you enjoying yourself and meeting some lads; it's time you had a decent social life.' Nicky made it sound as though I was a nun, but my life wasn't as quiet as that – just a lot calmer than hers. I had lots of friends, and I did go out a fair bit, but we weren't wild. That just wasn't in my nature.

I still lived with my mum, Pauline, and dad, Graham, in a house in the Leeds suburbs, the house we'd lived in since I was a baby. My big sister Tracy, who was five years older than me, had left home already. I'd been brought up in an environment where hard work and independence were thought of highly. My parents always had their own businesses, from an American-style car valeting service to a squash club, and, along with Tracy, I took all of that in from in an early age. I saw that if you were decent and worked hard, you could have a nice life. I knew that the holidays abroad and cars and house all came from the fact that my mum and dad were strong, committed people who did an honest day's work and put their family first.

To be honest, I'd had an idyllic childhood. I loved, and was good at, gymnastics and swimming. I liked horse riding as well, and I always had Tracy there beside me whatever I was doing, so I never felt lonely. We weren't spoiled – we were expected to do chores and be well-behaved – but Mum and Dad made sure we had a great time.

As I became a teenager, I never felt I had anything to rebel against, because I was really happy. Lots of people at school complained about their parents or home life, but I adored my family. Why would I want to do anything to hurt them? Besides, I didn't have the personality for rebellion. I liked things to be straightforward, predictable even, and it was that side of me that Nicky seemed determined to change.

That weekend, we hit Leeds. I was a bit nervous while I was getting ready. I remembered Nicky and her friends from college and they were so colourful and lively that I wondered whether I would fit in. I put on a pair of black trousers and a plain black top and left to meet them in town. It was a cold, wet night, but when I got there, they were all skimpily dressed as if it was the middle of summer.

'Going for a job interview later, Linz?' joked Nicky good-naturedly as soon as she saw my outfit. 'You're not exactly dazzling there, are you? I'm going to have my work cut out with you; come on, let's have a decent night for starters.' And we did.

It was the first of quite a few, as Nicky and I realized how well we got on. Every weekend we hit the clubs and bars, and Nicky always seemed to know where there was a party going on. After being quite nervous that first night, I started to enjoy myself. This group of girls always had a laugh; they chatted up lads and got plenty of attention, but they stuck together as well. Sometimes there were a few blokes in the gang – boyfriends or brothers or just friends – but it tended to be the girls who organized everything, and who made the most impact.

I fitted in much better than I'd expected, to tell the truth. Maybe at first I was a little resistant (perhaps I was just worried about spending too much money), but I loosened up pretty quickly after my initial reservations – you couldn't help do anything else when Nicky was around. After so many years with Dave, I was finally having the social life most other girls had been getting on with for a long time. Once Nicky came back into my life, she shook me up. She showed me how to be young and have a good time, and that was just what I needed.

She lived at home with her Mum on a council estate in Leeds, and most of their relatives seemed to have houses there as well. Nicky worked at another salon in the city centre, where she did really well with tips as the customers loved her personality, so she always had a bit of cash. We were completely different when it came to money. While Nicky was the type to spend her wages all in one go at the end of the week, I had my savings and I just couldn't bring myself to spend a fortune on clothes. Maybe the financial stability I'd learned from my parents made me that way; although they encouraged an entrepreneurial attitude, they also made sure that any risks were measured ones. I'd built up a little safety net for myself but spending £100 on a t-shirt, as Nicky would be quite happy to do, was way outside my comfort zone.

One Friday afternoon about a month after we'd met up again, Nicky popped into my work to confirm the arrangements for a new club that we were going to that night. 'We still on?' she checked. 'Course we are,' I replied. 'What are you wearing tonight?' she asked. I told her that I hadn't even thought about it, which was something Nicky couldn't begin to understand. 'Lindsey! That is why you always end up looking like you're going to a funeral! You've got a gorgeous figure –

why don't you show it off a bit for once?' That was a touchy subject for me. I was about 5 foot 4 inches and a size 8, but I'd always worried that I had a really big chest, so I tended to dress sensibly to cover myself up. 'I'm too self-conscious about my boobs. I don't want drunken men leering at me all night,' I told her. Predictably, she said, 'Show everyone what you've got, Linz. It's not your problem, it's theirs. Anyway, there's loads of us going tonight, so we can always protect you.' She mentioned the names of a few of the girls' current boyfriends before adding, 'And my little cousin Paul is going to drive us there – we'll save taxi money if he's driving, and we can always get him to be your bodyguard too.' With that, and a reminder to get to her house early so we could do each other's make-up, she left.

I got through my appointments that day – mostly nail extensions, which were starting to be very popular for the weekend and weddings – and thought that maybe Nicky was right, maybe I should dress a bit more like the rest of them. So that night, I took a sheer black top from my wardrobe and, instead of slipping a black t-shirt on underneath, I just wore a black bra. I was hardly half-naked, but to me, the outfit seemed pretty revealing.

I left my car at Nicky's house – I'd never even think of driving after a drink – and she clattered down the hall as soon as she heard me, tottering on heels she could barely walk in and poured into a top that she'd probably spent a fortune on earlier that day.

'God, Linz,' she said, pulling at my top, 'I can almost see a bit of flesh under there! You sure you're feeling all right?' Laughing, we went to her room to put the finishing touches to each other's make-up. I felt really happy that night – Nicky had given me a bit of confidence as she had dragged me to clubs and parties and shops over the past weeks, and it had definitely been for the best.

That night, another night out in town, promised to be a good one. We heard the front door downstairs slam as we were getting our bags ready, and Nicky's mum shouted. 'Nicky! Our Paul's here. You girls ready to go?' Nicky said that we would just be a minute and that her cousin Paul should wait outside for us. I was trying to loosen up, but there were always practicalities in my mind and I needed to ask Nicky a bit about this cousin of hers.

'This Paul. How young is he exactly?' I asked, worried that if he was her 'little' cousin he might not have a licence. Or insurance. Some habits are hard to break, and being sensible hadn't entirely been flushed out of my system.

'He's old enough, Linz,' she reassured me. 'Eighteen. Just three years younger than us.'

We walked out of her mum's front door towards a blue sports car waiting for us. I was trying to keep an open mind, but there was a skinny blond lad resting himself against the driver's door, smoking. I hated smoking. Absolutely hated it. 'All right girls?' he said as we walked over, casually flicking his fag butt away and breathing smoke in our faces.

'This is my mate, Lindsey,' said Nicky as we climbed in. Looking back, maybe there should have been a bolt of lightning or a peal of thunder. My future was starting there, that rainy night in Leeds. The reality was that I barely batted an eyelid. I just got in the back, and said 'Hiya'.

As we drove off, I noticed him having a sly look at me in his rear-view mirror. Actually, when I looked back at him I realized that he was quite good-looking. We caught each other's eyes in the mirror, noticed each other having a sly look, and he gave me a cheeky smile. I flushed a bit with embarrassment and looked out of the window.

'So, Lindsey,' he said – and at that moment I swear I could *hear* him smiling – 'Nicky tells me you're in beauty as well?'
'Yeah, that's right,' I told him. 'What is it you do for a living?'
He said he was a snooker player. What a ridiculous answer! 'Snooker?' I said to him. 'That's not a job, that's a hobby!' Actually, I knew already what he did as Nicky had told me, but I didn't want him to think I was bowled over by meeting him – her family all thought he was the bee's knees, but there was something about his cheeky confidence that made me want him to work a bit harder to impress me. He wasn't really on my radar, he'd barely registered, and I certainly didn't want to come across like an adoring fan. I didn't know anything about snooker anyway, and he seemed too young, too full of himself, too daft if he thought that hitting little balls into pockets with a stick was a real job. I had to stop myself giving him a lecture about setting up a pension early, but as I looked at him in the mirror again I saw that he was still smiling. He gave me a wink, a shrug, and got back to concentrating on the road – after he'd copped another look.

Paul dropped us off at the door of a new club that had just opened and went to park his car. It was loud and hot when we went in, but Nicky immediately spotted the rest of her crew and we went over to sit with them. We got some drinks and had a quick dance, and by the time we got back to the table, Paul was there. 'Lindsey!' he called, jokingly, 'I've missed you being so nice to me! Now I'm back, how about you give me a smile?' An 18-year-old like Paul Hunter just seemed like a kid to me, but I couldn't help but notice how attractive he was – for a kid.

My ex-boyfriend Dave was about my age, and I'd already decided that my next boyfriend would be older, very sensible, and probably somebody I could settle down with permanently. I wanted a stable relationship because that was what I'd grown up with. Although I enjoyed my nights out with Nicky – enjoyed them a lot – I still thought I'd be happiest sitting on the sofa, eating crisps and watching Saturday night telly. I wanted a boyfriend who would just as happily sit beside me rather than want to go out clubbing.

I had a great time that night. Nicky and I – and everyone else – got completely drunk and I almost forgot that I was dressed in a see-through top. I only remembered every time I caught Paul looking at me. Let him, I thought. He was just a lad, and he was the cousin of my best friend.

I left the club before him. Later that night, back home, I was a bit surprised when I found myself thinking about him. His smile kept popping into my head, and I realized that I was smiling myself when I pictured it.

I told myself it was the drink, tried not to worry about whether he'd driven himself home after all the vodka he'd packed away, and turned off my light.

My first night with Paul Hunter – and I hadn't a clue where it would all lead …

Chapter Three

Making an impression

Nicky and I kept in touch. We'd pop in to see each other at the salons where we worked, and we spoke on the phone most nights and went round to each other's houses quite often. She was soon planning another big night out, about a fortnight after the last one. This time there was a minibus organized to take a load of us to a club in Leeds and, despite myself, when Nicky said Paul would be there, I was looking forward to seeing him again. Nicky had told me that he often popped into her house as he was so close to her and her family, but so far he hadn't turned up when I was there. I hadn't seen him again since the night he had given us a lift into town. I didn't want to ask about him, as I wouldn't want to draw attention to the fact that I was a bit intrigued by him. Anyway, that didn't matter since my plan was to find Mr Sensible, wherever he might be, and Paul obviously wasn't him.

That night, I gave a bit of thought to how I was dressed. I put on quite a short skirt and a low-cut top. I'd given myself a facial and a manicure, and had taken care with my make-up. Of course, I didn't consciously do all this for Paul – it just so happened that this was a night when I felt I was looking good.

The minibus turned up at my house and Nicky bounded down the aisle to greet me as I stepped on. As she hugged me in her usual open way, I spotted Paul out of the corner of my eye sitting in an aisle seat. He nodded to me, with a smile on his face as usual, and I gave him a little smile back. It was only when I passed him to get to my seat beside Nicky that I noticed he wasn't alone. There was a dark-haired girl attached to him and, by the way she clung to his arm, they were obviously an item. It didn't stop Paul saying, 'All right, Lindsey?' as I went by. When I said I was fine, he added, 'Looking good, looking good!' It was dark so no one could see me blushing a bit, but I did notice that the girl beside him flashed me a look. Not a very friendly one at that.

'Who's that with your little cousin?' I asked Nicky once I'd sat down, trying to be as casual as possible.

'That's Gemma,' she whispered.

'Girlfriend?' I replied, in what I hoped was an offhand manner.

'Yeah,' she said, but after a bit of a pause.

I felt that I was on fairly safe ground here if I wanted to ask more questions. This was the sort of thing that came under the topic of us two just having a good old gossip. 'What's the story, then?' I asked.

'Well,' said Nicky, getting warmed up straight away, 'they've been together since school, really. She's a lovely girl, but they argue all the time. They often fall out before Paul goes away to tournaments and by the time he gets back, they've forgotten what they've argued about and get all loved up again. Paul's been around a bit but they always end up back together.'

'She's very pretty,' I said, and a voice in the back of my mind told me that if they'd been going out together since school, that wasn't very long as they were still just kids now.

'Isn't she?' answered Nicky, before going off onto another topic. I could hear her talking but, to my surprise, found that my mind had wandered back to the girl sitting beside Paul. She was kneeling on her seat, talking to someone behind her, and I could see that she really was pretty, with long hair and big brown eyes. She and Paul looked good together.

When we got to the club in town, everyone piled out of the minibus, paid their admission money, and went inside. As usual, Nicky and her friends made themselves at home by pulling lots of tables together and we all settled down in one place. There were long, velour couches against the back wall, with glass tables in front, and then individual chairs on the other side. I got myself a seat on one of the couches, quite a few spaces down from Paul and Gemma, and started drinking.

Before long, Gemma and Paul were arguing. Not loudly or badly, but enough that a few of us noticed. 'God, Paul,' shouted Nicky above the music. 'Do you two ever manage to get through a whole night without falling out?' She dragged me up to dance and by the time we got back, things seemed to have calmed down between Paul and Gemma – although only to the extent that they weren't talking at all.

I didn't know either of them particularly, so I couldn't make any judgement about what was going on, but I did think that I wouldn't be able to carry on like that if he was my boyfriend. I liked things settled and straightforward – I'd run a mile from complications. To be fair, neither of them seemed particularly bothered, which presumably meant that this was just a pattern for them. I didn't really care because I was having a good time with a few drinks inside me, and there were plenty of people to dance with.

The night went quickly, with nothing much different from any other night out, but at one point when I came back from the loo, I walked straight into the middle of Paul and his girlfriend having another of their rows. There were lots of hissed comments to each other as well as some shouting, and I slipped into my seat beside Nicky, who was watching it all with interest.

'Nicky,' I said, trying to get her attention away from the argument, 'do you think my skirt's too short?' 'Is that possible?' she said, glancing at it. 'Come on, Lindsey, you're young, you're gorgeous – stop worrying.' I tried to ignore the continued bickering from the side of me, at the same time as pulling my top further up and my skirt further down.

As I busied myself with my clothes, the very public, very heated row between Gemma and Paul ended with her storming off to dance without him. Nicky draped herself across me to talk to her cousin. 'Paul Hunter!' she said. 'When you two are like this, I can't believe you're supposed to be each other's first loves! You're on and off all the time! What's it about now?'

'Can't remember,' said Paul, despite the fact that the argument had still been going on minutes before. 'I've got other things on my mind.' With that, he leaned over to me, smiled a bit and said, 'Are there any more like you at home, but a bit younger?'

What a cheeky little rat! 'Are you saying that I'm nice but old?' I asked him. He looked at me all serious for a minute, then winked and went back to chatting to his friend on the other side.

Nicky was laughing, having heard it all, and I said to her, 'I feel self-conscious enough tonight about what I'm wearing without someone telling me I'm old as well!' She kept laughing and got me to have a giggle when she said, 'Oh, you're ancient, Linz, absolutely ancient! You should have said and you might have got a discount on your entry fee here – maybe they give cheap rates for pensioners!'

We all headed back to the minibus soon after. When Gemma got on, she made a point of not sitting beside Paul and I was left on my own when Nicky decided to go and keep him company. While I was sitting there, I kept thinking about what he had said to me – and every time I did, I couldn't help but smile. When I remembered Paul saying that I was looking good when I first got on the bus that night, I had an even bigger smile.

We all got dropped off at our houses in the early hours of the morning and when I got in, I couldn't stop thinking about what had happened that night. I knew it wasn't much, but Paul Hunter was so different to other boys that I had known that I had to admit he had made an impression on me. He was certainly on my radar now. I was used to Dave being attentive to me all the time, predictable even, but there was something about the way Paul had looked at me and joked with me that had already got under my skin. This was a boy with a lot of life in him – and that was something I was beginning to be drawn towards.

It was another few weeks before I met him again. Nicky and I were fast becoming best friends who wanted to meet up most nights. Neither of us could afford to go clubbing all the time, so we hung around each other's houses a lot; fortunately we both had friendly parents who always made us welcome.

All the Hunter cousins lived on the same estate and Paul and Nicky's family were especially close, going on holidays and for nights out together. She looked after him, and had done since they were kids; in turn, he adored her. He used to come round to Nicky's mum's house all the time and, over the next three or four months, I started to get to know him a bit better because of that. I'd be there to see Nicky, he'd pop round to see his cousin and auntie, and we'd just hang out together casually. He was still going out with Gemma – they'd got back together the day after falling out at that nightclub – and they were stuck in the pattern of falling out then making up over and over again.

I did like him – there was no doubt about that; and I was a bit attracted to him, I suppose, but I would have liked him anyway even without that. Paul was just great fun to be around. He lit up any room he was in, and everyone thought the world of him.

When he was round at Nicky's house, we'd all have a laugh

together. We'd watch films, eat loads, have a natter and muck about. Looking back on it, we weren't more than kids even though we were all working (I had to accept that snooker was a job now!), and we got into the habit of play fighting. Nicky and Paul would shove each other around, and I got drawn in. We spent hours in Nicky's bedroom or their front room rolling about the floor together, and, because they were family, I never thought much of it. I was close to Paul without there being any major stress on our blossoming relationship. In fact, I didn't even recognize it as that.

Away from Paul, I was having a great time with friends but I hadn't been seeing any particular lad seriously, preferring to just have a dance and a drink when I felt like it rather than rushing into another long-term relationship. On top of that, as I got to know Paul more and more, I was finding him easier and more fun to be around than any other boy I knew at that time. Because he was clearly still with Gemma despite their on-off behaviour, I could allow myself to have a little daydream about him without having to do anything about it, since he was spoken for.

One day, just as summer was beginning, I was round at Nicky's house. We were sitting out in the garden with her mum, having a nice cold glass of wine, when Nicky said, 'Here, Mum, tell Lindsey what you were talking about earlier.' Her mum shook her head and got the giggles, but it didn't stop Nicky. 'You like our Paul, don't you?' she asked. I tried to stay very nonchalant and said that I hadn't really thought about it, but they claimed it was obvious.

'Come on, Linz!' said Nicky, and she shoved me just the

way Paul did when we mucked about. 'What about all that play fighting you always do?' she asked. As she said that, Nicky kept pushing me just like Paul did, and I collapsed in a heap of giggles, knowing that she was right – we did that sort of thing a lot. 'But you do it too!' I protested. 'Yeah,' she admitted, 'but we do it because we've done it since we were kids – you and Paul do it because it's a chance to have a cuddle and a sly feel without admitting it!'

Slowly, it dawned on me that I did like him, but I didn't admit it to them. Not then.

How could I? He was still someone else's boyfriend.

Chapter Four

Golden boy

Sitting here amongst the packing boxes, I can't help but look at all the old photographs I come across. Memories can be tricky things – the same picture can bring back both good and bad. For me, looking at ones of Paul as a kid is somehow easier because I wasn't there. I wish I had seen every moment of his life, but photographs at least give me glimpses. I pick up one of him as a baby. The colour is fading and it looks older than it is; he's golden-haired and smiling, with his mum beside him, grinning as if she's going to burst with pride. I know that feeling.

Here's another of Paul at Christmas surrounded by people and presents, always smiling. Always smiling.

I pick up another. Paul looks tiny. A little boy dressed up like a man. He's wearing a waistcoat and bow tie, standing by a snooker table that seems made for a giant. His parents have told me the stories behind these images, and Paul has gone over his memories too. I feel as if they are my memories now – I'll be the one to pass them on to our baby girl when she grows up. They are evidence of how handsome he was, how talented, and how adored. I wasn't the only one to fall in love with Paul Hunter.

Once I got to know Paul and his family, I found out that he could always make people fall in love with him. It wasn't a manipulative thing; he didn't explicitly decide to have people fall at his feet so that he could get what he wanted – it was just that he was incredibly engaging. Paul would do anything for anyone and most people would do anything for him too. I remember thinking at the time, What's going on here? Why am I suddenly head over heels for this boy? Of course, it wasn't sudden really but I was still shocked by it.

I suppose I was becoming part of Paul's world without it being a big deal. If I had been his girlfriend at that stage, I'm not sure that I would have got to know him as well as I did. We spent our first months together quite naturally, with no pressure, and that would always stand us in good stead. As time went on, I found out a lot about his background and it helped me make sense of some of his behaviour.

To be honest, Paul had never really grown up.

We had been brought up very differently as children. Both sets of parents are still together – in itself, quite unusual nowadays, I guess – but snooker-mad Paul was treated like a little prince from the moment he was born, whereas my mum and dad showed their love by giving me strong values and independence.

Paul's big sister Leanne had been born three years before him in 1975, the same year as me. His mum, Kristina, was over the moon when she got pregnant with Paul – he was very much a wanted child – but she had a huge scare when she started bleeding very heavily at three months and thought she was having a miscarriage. Paul's dad, Alan, and a friend carried her upstairs to bed feet first to try and stop her losing so much blood, but I know that it was terrifying – she was sure she'd lose the baby. Next day, she was taken to hospital and stayed there for a week. When the bleeding stopped and she was sent home, she says she somehow knew that her baby was a survivor, and the rest of the pregnancy was fine.

Alan was present at the birth and seemingly was so overcome by it all that as soon as the baby came out and the doctor said, 'It's a boy!' the proud new dad keeled over in a faint.

Paul Alan Hunter was born on 14 October 1978, weighing 5lbs 3oz. He was put in an incubator for a few days as he was so tiny, and when his mum looked at him, he seemed like a little dolly; perfect and with incredibly blond, almost silvery-white, hair. He liked attention from the outset – and that wasn't to change much. When you put baby Paul down, he'd scream. If you picked him up, he'd smile. Everyone says that, as a baby, he just wanted a cuddle and a bit of love.

He had an extended family nearby, with several cousins who were roughly the same age as him, and Polish grandparents, Babcia and Dziadek, on his mum's side. Everyone loved the golden-haired little boy who had come into the family. However, more than anything, Paul was a mummy's boy. He hated Kristina going out, and whenever she did, he would sulk at the bottom of their stairs; often he got his own way and made his mum feel so guilty that she would come back early.

This didn't stop in later years. When Paul was about 13, his mum came home to find him asleep on the sofa one night. She tried to wake him up, but nothing worked – he was so sound asleep that prodding and whispering in his ear had no effect whatsoever. Finally, she lugged her teenage son upstairs and tucked him up in bed without disturbing his dreams. It was years and years later that Paul admitted to her that he was awake the whole time and only pretending to be asleep so that she would cuddle him, pamper him, and make him feel like her baby again.

Any of the tricks Paul played, however, were purely fun and games. He got away with a lot because he was a genuinely nice lad who had a smile to break hearts and a sense of humour that got him through everything. Even as we faced our darkest days together, that smile would appear and the sense of humour would kick in and I sometimes got glimpses of the little boy he must have been. He was a crowd-pleaser even as a kid; a soft touch who always did his best to keep everyone happy, and who wanted everyone to like him.

These days, as I sit without him, I wish I could go back to the years when I didn't know him. I want to soak up all those memories, those times when I wasn't in his life. I wish I could just top myself up on all the Paul days to keep me going. I'm sure if I had known him then, he'd have made me adore him then too. Before his true talent came out, Kris and Alan say that they had no idea what he would become but they always had a feeling that the smiling little lad with the golden hair would capture many more hearts than just those of his immediate family.

By the time Paul turned three in October 1981, he had already started showing an interest in snooker. He kept trying to hit marbles with a chopstick so when Christmas came, a tiny snooker table was bought. This was at the time when snooker was reaching its heyday – it was on telly a lot and there were some real characters associated with the game so there was always some sort of coverage going on. Paul was born in the year that the BBC first decided to give blanket coverage to the World Championship. Snooker was booming when the little boy got his first taste of life on the baize.

On Christmas morning 1981, Paul opened the miniature snooker set and it was pretty much the only thing he played with all day long. It was so small that it fitted onto the coffee table in the lounge, but it was big enough to start turning Paul's dreams into reality. He picked up that snooker cue when he was three and never really put it down again.

For his fifth birthday, Paul was given a 6ft x 3ft set, which was kept in the living room, and it was his favourite possession. Alan played regularly with friends at a local club called Snooker 2000. One night, when Paul was eight, Alan's usual partner rang to say that he couldn't make the game that night. As he put the telephone down and shouted through to tell Kristina what was going on, young Paul jumped up and down by his side. 'Dad! Dad!' he shouted. 'Take me! Take me!' Alan tried to ignore him, but an excitable Paul wasn't too easy to shut out. He wouldn't stop pleading for Alan to take him to the snooker club, and his dad finally said that, if it was up to him he would, but the manager would never let a kid in to play. He hoped that would be an end to the matter, but he should have known Paul wouldn't be put off so easily.

'Dad! Dad!' he went on. 'Can we find out? Can we ask if they'll let me in? Please, Dad? Please?' Alan relented. Given that he was pretty confident that he was right and Paul wouldn't get to play, it seemed easier to make the trip and let someone else explain things to his snooker-mad son. When they got there, either the snooker gods were watching or the manager was in a particularly good mood because Paul got his way and he was allowed to play his dad on a proper-sized snooker table in a proper club.

The boy was like a duck to water.

He never looked back.

Paul and his dad went to Snooker 2000 a few times over the next couple of weeks, and it amazed everyone there that the little lad was giving his father such a good game. People used to congregate while he was at the table, until there were dozens standing watching. He was cute – which helped – but he could also play the game, which made things even better.

Now snooker is a pricey hobby and Alan was renowned for being careful with cash so everyone assumed Paul would just have to accept that the 6ft x 3ft table in the living room was going to have to do for now. They hadn't accounted for the attention Paul had been getting while he was playing his dad. The club decided that he was so good for business that they would let him play for free as often as he liked, and Paul was over the moon.

When he was 10, Alan took little Paul to the Crucible in Sheffield, the sport's most famous venue, for the first time.

There the boy made a wish that would come true sooner than anyone thought: 'One day, Dad,' he said, 'one day, I'd love to play here.' He knew what he wanted from that moment on.

Paul's first love was just playing the game. He wasn't bothered about competitions and trophies to begin with, but it soon became clear that he was so talented, such challenges were the next logical step. He was winning under-12 tournaments from when he was 10 – the same age that he first beat his dad at the Snooker 2000 club. He was 11 years and one week old when he made his first century break (scoring more than a hundred points in one break).

Of course, he lost sometimes. He entered a Prestatyn Pontins under-16s tournament when he was only 10 and was devastated to lose in the second round. He rushed back to the chalet he'd been sharing with his dad, absolutely heartbroken. In later years, fellow players and fans would all say that you could never tell if Paul had won or lost a game because he always had the same happy demeanour. This certainly wasn't the case when he was 10. He sobbed his heart out and said to Alan over and over again, 'You said I had a chance! You said I had a chance!' It was the last time he ever got really emotionally upset about losing; he was never up or down from that point on. Snooker was massively important to him but there was a dividing line, and that first clear loss was the turning point. He learned. He learned that you couldn't always trust your talent – luck was involved. He learned that you don't make yourself feel any better by getting upset. He learned that there's always another game just around the corner. As

Paul matured he was gracious in success and defeat, and he never had a bad word to say about anybody.

He was never sulky about the game but he was extremely competitive. Snooker was more than a hobby for Paul – it was a calling. Just before his 12th birthday, he moved from Snooker 2000. He was asked to bring his talent and potential elsewhere – he was poached, really – by the management at The Manor, a health and leisure centre that also had a snooker club. That was where the 1986 World Champion Joe Johnson practised. Joe was never Paul's coach but he did take him under his wing to an extent and gave him advice on shot selection, as well as no doubt telling him plenty of stories about life in the snooker world.

Paul beat Joe for the first time when he was 13 years old, and that year he also won his first prize money at a Willie Thorne under-16s competition in Leicester. The prize was £100 and he got an extra £25 for the highest break as well. From this age on he was pretty much self-financing.

Kristina was more sceptical about the whole business than Alan. His dad went with Paul to the club and games, so he knew what was going on and how good Paul was. However, Kris tended not to be there, so she only heard about it all second hand. Maybe you wouldn't really appreciate how good your kid was at something like that at such a young age unless you were seeing the proof for yourself. Kris tried hard to get him to go to school and do his homework but Paul couldn't have been less interested. Many mornings he'd get dropped off at school, only to nip off to his grandparents, Babcia and Dziadek, for the day to get spoiled rotten. He'd be treated like royalty before slinking back to school to get picked up again by his unsuspecting mother later in the day. By the time Paul was 14, he was allowed to leave school by the education authorities on one condition – he had to employ a private tutor. From that point on, Paul had nothing to distract him from his beloved game.

Once her son started to earn money, Kristina realized that what Alan was telling her and what she hoped was true wasn't just parental pride – Paul Hunter really was going to be snooker's next big thing. All he wanted was to play, all the time, in whatever tournament he could.

He won the Pontins under-16 tournament at the age of 14, which sent out a message to the sport. It was a really prestigious event that had been won by lots of lads who have gone on to become famous names in snooker, such as Stephen Hendry. When Paul won, they all knew that here was someone who would be a danger to them in a few years' time. He hadn't had coaching up until that point – Paul always said that while coaching might work for some people, he thought that most problems needed to be dealt with in your own head. It certainly worked for him, but he was very young to be hanging around snooker tournaments and halls all the time.

People have this image of snooker being played in smoky, dingy places, real men's clubs, with an atmosphere of drinking and being a right lad – and that's exactly what it was like when Paul was learning his trade. I've heard from his friends that there were always girls hanging around. As a result, he definitely grew up quickly – perhaps too quickly. He lost his virginity at a very young age – well before it was legal. He definitely had an eye for the ladies, although I don't like to dwell on it now.

The first time Alan took her boy away for a week, Kristina felt as if her heart had broken. He turned pro and went to the Norbreck Castle in Blackpool, to what is known as 'qualifying school'. There, between three and four hundred budding players were competing for the glory of reaching the televised stages of tournaments. Paul's talent shone through and he won all of his first 36 matches as a professional. Then when he was 16, they went away to a tournament for a whole month. It was a great adventure for Paul, of course, but Kris was very aware that she was losing her smiling little mummy's boy. Eventually, she says, she got used to him being gone for periods of time.

Of course, she never dreamed for a moment how soon he would be gone from her life forever.

Chapter Five

Summer 1997

When Paul and I started seeing each other at Nicky's house, I didn't think of him as drop–dead gorgeous – I liked him purely based on how cheeky and funny he was. He was tall and wore his blond hair in what I called 'curtains' – short at the back and floppy over each side of his forehead. It was very much a young boy's style – a bit of a state really. He wasn't bothered about clothes or fashion, and usually just wore a jumper and jeans.

The other part of his life took place in snooker halls and exhibition centres up and down the country, and often abroad. Most snooker players take a long break during the summer, but they often do exhibition matches or corporate events to boost their income even when there aren't any actual tournaments going on. Nicky showed me lots of photographs of Paul in his snooker gear, standing beside tables, or shaking hands with dignitaries presenting prizes, and I found it hard to reconcile that image with the daft teenager who would push me onto the sofa and tickle me until I cried tears of laughter. Sometimes I would read his name in the sports pages of papers and he seemed like a different person in a different world. He was playing snooker all the time in those early days. As soon as he had turned professional at the age of 16, he had caused a sensation at the UK Championships by beating Alan McManus, the world number six, in the first round by 9–4. That was an amazing achievement and really put Paul on the map. He had followed it up by becoming the youngest player to reach the semi-finals of a ranking event in the 1996 Regal Welsh Open, when he was just 17. In that same year, he also reached the last eight of the UK Championships, where he beat some big names including Willie Thorne; in fact, he played a great game, but lost to Stephen Hendry who eventually won the whole tournament.

It was as if Paul had two lives at the time I met him – the professional international snooker player and the 18-year-old boy. In fact, because he was locked away in the snooker world when he was playing, he was really immature on a lot of levels. When he and Nicky and I mucked about, it allowed him to let off steam and be a kid again. Maybe he needed to do that since his actual childhood had been spent in a man's world; maybe he wanted to stay a child just a bit longer.

Still, when all was said and done, he was a lad – and lads are only happy tickling girls for so long before they start to think of other things! One night we were at Paul's mum and dad's house where he still stayed, and his cousin Anthony had come along as well. I'd been there a couple of times before, as a friend of Nicky's more than anything, and I'd met Alan and Kris briefly. Paul got us all a drink from the cabinet – he was knocking back a huge amount of vodka as usual – and we settled down to watch a video. It was a boring film, and everyone started to get a bit restless.

Paul suggested, 'Let's have a game of truth or dare.' Well, I wasn't that naive; in my experience truth or dare was usually an excuse for a good snog. I have to admit that I was hoping we'd get a chance, so I didn't mind at all. By the time it was my turn, Paul made it clear that he'd be asking the questions. 'Truth or dare, Linz?' he said, with a smile. I went for truth, no doubt as everybody expected me to – I wasn't going to risk a dare because it could have been anything! 'Right,' said Paul, with a twinkle in his eye. 'Is it true that you're absolutely dying to kiss me?'

Anthony and Nicky both burst out laughing as my cheeks reddened. 'Absolutely not!' I said. Paul waggled his finger in my face. 'Lindsey Fell,' he mocked, 'I think you're lying. You have not told the truth, so it is within my powers to make you do a dare.' I made a face that was meant to look completely unconcerned as he continued: 'As you lied so disgracefully about the fact that you are desperate to get your hands on me, I have to make the punishment fit the crime.' He was really getting into this now. 'So – I dare you to give Paul Hunter the best snog he has ever had in his life, and ignore Anthony and Nicky if they try to stop you.'

I was sitting beside Paul on the sofa while he made his announcement, so I wiggled a bit closer. I knew that I was going to do it, and I was looking forward to the look on everyone's faces afterwards. As I moved closer to him, Paul took my hand and leaned in towards me, kissing me first. Given that it was my dare, he was putting in a lot of the work. We both got into it pretty quickly, while Nicky and Anthony shouted in the background: 'You two can stop any minute, you know. Don't feel obliged to keep going. Give your tongues a rest!' It was all a laugh and nothing serious, but it did change things to the extent that we both knew there hadn't been any hardship in kissing each other; in fact, it was just wonderful.

The rest of the night was pretty unremarkable. Paul and Anthony gave each other drinking dares while Nicky and I giggled about what had just happened. Nicky and Anthony were staying over at Paul's that night, so I ordered a taxi to pick me up. As I left, Nicky gave me a cuddle but I was a bit disappointed that Paul didn't say anything else. However, just as I got into the cab he flew out of his front door. I rolled my window down. 'Here, Lindsey,' he said, 'I just wanted to let you know if you ever fancy another game of truth or dare, well – I'm your man.' He gave me a wink and went back inside, leaving me thinking nice thoughts about him all the way home.

I didn't see Paul for about a week or so after that, and it gave me time to think. I realized that I did find him cheeky but so lovely with it that I couldn't help but like him. I kept asking Nicky what was going on between Paul and Gemma, but it obviously made her a bit uncomfortable. 'Look, Lindsey,' she said one day, 'I know that you and Paul get on really well, and

I know you like each other, but he's still with Gemma. They've been together for so long that they're pretty much an established couple. There's nothing I'd like better than for you two to start going out together, but I don't think it'll happen, not while Gemma's around.'

While the penny dropped for me and I had to admit that I was interested in him, Paul was still committed to another girl. Every now and again, when he was on a break from her, we'd go for a meal, or into a club in town, usually with other people, and we almost always ended up having a kiss at the end of the night. After about six weeks of this, I felt as though we were getting closer, but I realized that he was still seeing Gemma. I'd never even spoken to the girl, other than to say 'hiya' if she was in our crowd, but I did spend a lot of time thinking about her.

My relationship with Dave had been very straightforward: we liked each other, we went out with each other, and we were nice to each other. I knew that I was naive and a bit old-fashioned, but I thought that partners should be faithful to each other. Every time Paul and I kissed, I felt a twinge of discomfort because I knew he would probably soon be going back to Gemma.

One night, we were in his car after a meal out. I'd taken my car too, so it was quite clear that I wasn't angling to get a lift home; we were there for a bit of a kiss and cuddle as usual. After he'd been kissing me for what seemed like hours, and I'd been warding off his wandering hands for just about the same amount of time, Paul suddenly pulled away from me. 'Lindsey Fell,' he said, looking into my eyes, 'I can't decide whether to think of you as the world's biggest tease, or as a challenge.' In the life he led on the snooker circuit, he was used to women just falling into bed with him straight away. There were always girls hanging around the tournaments and snooker halls – snooker groupies really – and Paul wasn't shy about the fact that he had an eye for the ladies.

He always met a girl, slept with her on the first night, and that was it. Meanwhile, I'd only ever slept with Dave and we'd been together for six years! 'Well, Paul,' I told him, 'maybe you shouldn't think of me as either of those. Maybe you should just get it into your head that not all girls throw their knickers away on the first date!'

'First date? First date?' he screeched, with the usual twinkle in his eyes. 'It's been going on a lot bloody longer than a first date, Linz!' I don't think that Paul ever understood that for me to consider sleeping with a second person was a big deal. I'd always thought I'd be with Dave forever. It was actually quite unsettling for me to think I'd ever have to have sex with someone else. 'You are kidding, Lindsey,' he said. 'You're actually saying "no"? And meaning it?' He seemed shocked that I wouldn't have sex with him, but I was just as shocked that some girls would sleep with boys who weren't even their proper boyfriends. We were complete opposites there.

'Yes, I mean it,' I told him. 'And there's something else I want to talk about.' He got that uncomfortable look in his eye that blokes always seem to get when girls say they want to talk about things. 'Gemma. What's going on there, Paul? I want to know where I stand. Is she your girlfriend or am I?'

Paul actually looked a bit flustered for a moment. I'd assumed that he was almost doing it deliberately – stringing two girls along at the same time – but he claimed otherwise. 'It's not as clear cut as you think, Lindsey,' he said. 'I don't think it's clear cut at all, Paul,' I told him. 'I think it's very messy and I'm not happy with it.'

He pulled away from me and sat back in the driver's seat. 'I wouldn't choose for things to be like this,' he answered. 'It's just that Gemma and I, we have a history together. She's been my girlfriend since school – you know I left at 14, Lindsey; she was my only bit of reality sometimes when I came back from tournaments. She was just a girl who'd been to school with me and, if I'd been here all the time and having a normal life, we probably would have had a normal relationship. But something's gone odd – we spend all our time rowing.'

'So? Make a decision, Paul,' I said. 'This hasn't really got anything to do with snooker, has it? You just need to decide whether you want her or me, and then act on it.'

'There's more to it than that,' he replied. 'She really loves me. We go back a long way. I don't like to hurt her.'

'But you're happy to hurt me instead?'

'Of course not. But you're so different. You're independent and you don't run after me.' He moved over to give me another kiss. 'If we fell out, you'd just drive off on your own, wouldn't you?'

'Too right I would,' I said. 'And don't think your little speech is going to get me into bed either,' I joked, although secretly I was falling for him big time and was considering whether to take it a stage further. That night ended like lots of other nights – we had a bit more kissing and cuddling, Paul tried to move it on, and I eventually left to drive home alone to my mum and dad's house.

This went on for another few weeks until one day in the late summer of 1997 Nicky asked if I would like to go on a last-minute holiday with her and her mum. I jumped at the chance – a week on a Spanish beach sounded perfect to me. We could sunbathe all day and enjoy ourselves all night. I told her I'd love to go and she set about making the arrangements.

Only a couple of days after she'd first discussed it, Nicky had the holiday booked. She never wasted any time once she got something into her head. I went round to her house one night after work so we could start packing and get ourselves organized.

'Here,' said Nicky, as we wrote out our lists, 'I've got something to tell you.' She had her back to me as she said it so I couldn't read her face. 'Our Paul's decided that he's coming too – maybe you'll finally decide that you're right for each other.' I hadn't seen that one coming. 'He's coming on holiday with us?' I paused to think about this. 'Well, it doesn't really matter – I don't think Paul feels that way, Nicky,' I told her. 'He doesn't seem to be able to make up his mind about Gemma. I don't even know when they're on and when they're off these days.'

Nicky went quiet, and I had to ask: 'He's back on with Gemma again, isn't he?' She nodded. 'Yeah, he is; he was on the phone to her last night when he was round here. Think about it though, Linz – if he was crazy about her why would he want to go on holiday with you?'

'He's going on holiday with *you*, Nicky; you're his family. I'm just someone who happens to be there. I'm all right for a kiss and a cuddle, but not good enough for him to dump Gemma properly.' I sounded a bit bitter, which was exactly how I felt. The cheek of him, I thought. He'd been trying to get me to sleep with him and yet he was back again with his girlfriend.

'I think he has tried to break it off with her, but he's finding it really hard. Gemma isn't one to give up easily. If it's any consolation, babes, we think he's mad and he should go for you,' she said, supportively.

It seemed to me that even though Paul and I kissed every now and again, and although I did think he was interested, that was that. I felt a bit angry with him. Did he think I was going to be some little holiday fling? Did he think we would sleep together out there and then he would come back to Gemma? If he did, he didn't know me very well at all. When I went home that night, I made a decision.

I was sure that I would have a great time with Nicky.

I was even more sure that I wouldn't let Paul Hunter ruin my holiday.

Chapter Six

Summer love

I didn't see Paul again before we left, so it was only when my dad dropped me off at the airport to meet the others that I had a chance to reflect on my decision. I may have decided that I wouldn't let him affect me, but I hadn't been prepared for how he seemed more good-looking every time I saw him. Paul wasn't one to hold a grudge either. As soon as I walked into the terminal pulling my little case on wheels, he ran over, took it out of my hand and gave me a cuddle. 'All right, Lindsey?' he asked. 'Ready to show Spain what having a good time looks like?' I just laughed, glad that he had such an easy way about him. I never wanted us to fall out and, to be honest, we hadn't (it would take a lot to make Paul fall out with anyone), but I had been worried that there might have been a bit of bad feeling between us after I'd brought up the subject of Gemma.

On the holiday, it was Nicky, Paul, her mum and me. We'd rented an apartment only a few minutes from the beach. It had three bedrooms, one for Nicky and me, one for her mum, and one for Paul. I think the arrangement was meant to give us some privacy but we didn't need it – we all knew each other so well by now that we were happy to spend a whole week together. It wasn't as if we needed separate bedrooms for bringing anyone back either – Nicky wasn't exactly on the pull with her mum there, and I had no intention of letting Paul break down my defences.

The holiday was an absolute blast. We all knew that we only had seven days to enjoy ourselves and we were ready to make every minute count. From the first day, it was obvious that Paul and Gemma were back on again. He kept going off to call her every few hours, which I thought was a bit odd. It wasn't like a lad to be so worried, and I felt that it was further proof that he just wasn't interested in me any more. Nicky soon put another idea in my head, though. 'It's not him who's worried about Gemma,' she said. 'It's her who's worried about you being here. She'll be sitting at home thinking of you in a bikini and Paul seeing you every minute. I bet she's asked him to check in every so often every day.'

We fell into a pattern straight away. Nicky's mum got friendly with some other women in the apartment complex, so the three of us would all go clubbing until about 3am or 4am every night. We'd stagger back to our rooms, and fall out of bed quite early so that we could sleep off the hangovers on the beach the next day. Paul was still calling Gemma a lot but it didn't really bother me. I felt I understood the situation better, that they were obviously quite solid together, so I concentrated on enjoying myself.

After a few days, we started chatting to another group of

holidaymakers from Manchester who were staying near us. There were a few lads who weren't attached to any of the girls in their group, and they were a good laugh. Paul didn't make it down to the beach one day as he was so drunk from the night before, and, by the time he did, Nicky and I were mucking about with the Manchester boys. As Paul came down the steps to the beach, he looked furious. He sat beside all of us on a deckchair but he didn't join in any of the laughs. After a while, he got up, went back to the apartment and didn't come back.

Nicky went to check on him at one point. When she came back, she said, 'He's really pissed off that you're talking to these boys, Linz. When I asked him to come back, he said he didn't want to watch you flirting and flaunting yourself at strangers all day!'

'Is he joking?' I asked her. 'He's not my boyfriend – he's the one mucking me about, so why should he get a say in how I behave?' Nicky ran back to the apartment again to speak to Paul, and I shouted after her, 'And tell him I am not flirting … or flaunting!'

When Nicky returned, she said that he was pretending to sleep but she reckoned he was probably watching us all from the apartment window. I cranked it up a notch then and laughed as loud as I could as one of the boys threw me into the little kiddie pool on the beach. If Paul was watching, that would give him something to think about – this was exactly the sort of mucking around we had done together before we started kissing and cuddling earlier in the year.

I wasn't prepared for the effect it would have.

The next person to come down the steps to the beach was Nicky's mum. She'd gone back to the apartment after doing a bit of shopping and when she saw him, she asked Paul why he was looking so miserable. He must have laid it on thick because she obviously felt sorry for him. 'That poor boy!' she said. 'Do you know that our Paul is trying to get an early plane home, Lindsey, because he's so upset at you looking to get another boyfriend right under his nose? He can't stand seeing you with other boys, love.'

I was speechless! Almost.

'What?' I said, really offended that I was being portrayed as the villain here. 'He's the one with a girlfriend! He's either seeing me or he's not – and I thought he wasn't.'

It turned out that Paul couldn't get an early flight back to Leeds anyway, but he still acted as if there was a huge drama going on – he locked himself in his room for the rest of the day in a huff. I didn't know what to make of all this. We hadn't spoken about 'us' all holiday, we'd just had a laugh. Anyway – was there an 'us'? I had no idea.

He didn't come out clubbing with us that night but Nicky had told him where we were going. Paul showed up after an hour or so and we all danced and drank as if nothing had happened. On the way back to the apartment, he pulled me behind and took my hand without saying anything. We just walked together in silence for a while. My heart was fluttering even though I was still angry with him for putting the blame on me. We fell further and further behind Nicky, and then Paul stopped. He pulled me towards him, and I thought my heart was going to fly out of my chest.

'Lindsey,' he said softly into my ear, 'I don't know what's going on. Do you?'

'I've got even less of a clue than you, Paul,' I told him. 'I'm not attached to anyone else. I'm a free agent. You're the one who has to make a decision.'

'When I'm with you, everything else goes away. I can be myself. When it's just us, it's fantastic – but when I see Gemma, I get confused.'

'It doesn't have to be confusing, Paul,' I told him. 'It's pretty straightforward. Just decide. Make your own mind up. Don't be influenced by anybody else. Don't …' I had to stop because he was kissing me. He felt so open to me that night. He wasn't putting on a show for anyone, he was being completely honest. The problem was that he was always trying to keep other people happy – and in the process ended up making himself unhappy.

That warm Mediterranean night, we kissed and held each other for what seemed like forever. Paul pressed himself against me and I knew what he wanted to happen next, but I couldn't do it. I wouldn't sleep with him while everything was still uncertain. I'd only known him for about five months, and although that might be ages for some people, I'd had years with Dave and only Dave. I wasn't going to fall into bed without some guarantee.

We walked back to the apartment. Even though we were going to sleep in the same apartment, it would be in different beds. 'Lindsey,' Paul said just as we opened the door. 'It's you, Lindsey, I want to be with you.' I could feel all the hairs on my arms stand up as he said it. 'I'm going to finish with

Gemma once and for all. As soon as we get back to Leeds, that's it. Then, you and me – we're a couple.' He kissed me again and poked me in the ribs, smiling. 'You can't hold out forever, Lindsey – look at me. I'm bloody irresistible!'

For the last bit of the holiday, everything was perfect. I told Nicky what had happened, and she acted as if we'd just announced that we'd won the lottery. Paul and I spent all our time together after that, but I still kept it to kissing and cuddling. He was right – to me, he was irresistible. I couldn't help myself. It was as if I had turned a corner and noticed what was there all along – I was besotted. I wouldn't let Paul know that though – not yet!

The flight back to Leeds was uneventful but, for me, there was a feeling that something important was about to happen. Paul and I smiled at each other a lot, and Nicky grinned like a Cheshire cat. I knew that the pattern with Gemma and Paul falling out and making up wasn't going to be an easy one to break, and I might need patience. He'd tried to end it with her before, but now that he had definitely decided that he wanted me, he had a focus. I didn't feel badly that he was breaking up with her because I'd asked him to. They didn't seem to be making each other happy and hadn't for a long time, so they were both going to be better off apart.

When we got off the plane, I told Paul that I would speak to him the following weekend. I didn't want to be chasing him up every day asking if he had finished with Gemma yet. He'd said he would do it and that was good enough for me. I wanted to give him a bit of space and some time to think about his decision, and then the chance to carry it through the best way he saw fit.

I came out of the arrivals gate and saw Mum and Dad waiting for me with big smiles on their faces. I'd missed them just as much as they'd missed me. Paul had met them informally a few times when he'd picked me up from home, or when he was hanging around with Nicky, but he was just one of the gang then. Now, he was my boyfriend-to-be. As everyone greeted each other, I had an idea.

I wasn't the kind of girl to have temporary boyfriends, and if Paul was to be my official boyfriend there was something he'd have to do for me. I'd been with Dave for years and part of the reason that worked was that he got on so well with my mum and dad. It was obvious: it was time for Paul to meet my parents properly.

Chapter Seven

My world

I got through the week at work somehow, and only spoke to Nicky on the phone. We didn't go out anywhere as we were both short of funds after the holiday. I didn't ask her how she thought Paul was getting on, but she did say that while he was round at her house he didn't call Gemma at all. I wasn't too worried anyway. It had always been my philosophy that it's useless to waste time worrying about things you can't change, and this was no exception. I was mad about Paul but if he didn't split up with Gemma, that was his choice and I'd just have to learn to live with it.

However, on Saturday morning the telephone rang at just after seven o'clock. It was Paul, and he could hardly contain himself. 'Lindsey!' he shouted. 'I did it. I finished with Gemma!' I was delighted, but it was early and he'd caught me unawares. 'Oh, Paul, that's fantastic, babes – did you have to let me know so early though?' He said that he'd been keen to let me know before I went to work so he'd set his alarm. This was impressive stuff from the boy who could sleep for

England. Mind you, I didn't fool myself – he'd go back to bed for the rest of the day while I did the Saturday brides.

We arranged that he'd meet me from work that night, and when he hung up, I was so excited I could barely get ready. 'Who was that on the phone?' Mum asked when I went down for breakfast. 'Oh, that was Paul,' I told her. 'Nicky's cousin?' 'Yeah,' I said nonchalantly. 'What did he want at this time of the morning?' asked Mum, confused. 'We were just working out what time to meet tonight.' Mum said something about how nice it was that we all got on so well together and I mentioned – very casually! – that it would just be me and Paul going out. That got her attention. 'Didn't I say? Paul's my boyfriend now.' I thought that would work and it did. 'Oh, Lindsey – you'll have to bring him round for Sunday lunch! Next week – how does that sound? We'll have to get to know the lad a bit better,' she said and went off to tell my dad.

I got through the day with a knot of excitement in my stomach and changed in the back room of the salon before Paul arrived to meet me. I saw him through the front window of the shop and he was just gorgeous. And mine, I thought to myself. When I went out, he gave me a big kiss and cuddle and we headed off for a few drinks in town before going to an Italian restaurant for a lovely meal. He wasn't too keen to talk about how things had gone with Gemma so I didn't press him, and I decided to break the other news to him once he'd got a bit tipsy.

'What are you doing next Sunday, Paul?' I asked.

'Nothing. Why?'

'Oh, it's just that Mum and Dad want you to come round

for your Sunday lunch.' As I said it, the colour seemed to drain from his face.

'Lunch with Big Bad G?' he asked. It was a nickname that he'd decided on for my dad from when we all first started hanging around together. Dad wasn't that big and he certainly wasn't bad, but Paul seemed to think that he was some sort of cartoon character always on the lookout for anyone who might mess with his girls.

'Paul!' I reprimanded. 'Stop calling him that! He's just my dad.'

'Yeah – but I'm the one hanging around Graham Fell's precious little girl,' he replied. 'He could kill me, you know.'

'My mum and dad are so laid back; you've got no worries there, they're lovely people. As long as I'm happy, they'll be happy.'

He was still uptight. 'God, Linz,' he said. 'Will I have to use lots of different knives and forks? Will there be loads of different cutlery? And what will the food be like? Will I want to eat it – is it fancy? And will it all be in bowls and I'll have to help myself? Can you fill my plate for me, Linz, just in case I spill stuff? And can you shove the cutlery towards me that I'm meant to use?'

I couldn't really understand what he was on about but he did seem genuinely worried, not just winding me up. What was the problem? 'It's just that you've been brought up so differently to me, Lindsey,' he explained. 'Your family life, your parents, your background – it's not what I'm used to and it makes me nervous.'

Was that it? Did he think he'd make a fool of himself? And

did he think my parents were the sort who'd be so shallow that they wouldn't like him if he used the wrong knife? I suppose, like most kids, I'd always assumed that I had the same life as anyone else, the same type of parents and the same luck. As I got older, I realized that I had been wrong to think this.

Actually, I was the luckiest girl in the world. From the moment I screamed my first scream in August 1975, I was at the heart of a family so loving and so strong, they would give me all the ammunition I would ever need to cope with life. Mum and Dad have always said that they never brought us up in any special way. They didn't sit down and work out a plan for raising two daughters; they just did their best and they never lifted a hand to either of us. We always did as we were told, but that was out of respect and knowing the difference between right and wrong.

My childhood was such a solid time. We always sat down for meals together and talked. Every Friday, Tracy and I would have a bath and then snuggle up in our dressing gowns. A table would be pulled into the lounge and we'd all eat a proper three-course meal together and chat about our week. I know that what they were doing was teaching us to eat properly as much as anything; but to Tracy and me it was just a lovely cosy way of ending the week. We were like a little gang.

Tracy and I have always been close. She says she loved me from the moment she set eyes on me as a new baby. We look alike but our personalities are different, though. I'm more like my dad – we're quite calm, we don't really like arguments, and when we think we're right, we stick to our guns. Tracy is like Mum – they're pretty fiery, they will argue and they will cry and shout, but they calm down again just as quickly. Both of us were independent and learned from an early age to stand on our own two feet.

One place we learned independence was on family holidays abroad. We often went to Cala d'Or, in Majorca, where a business friend of my parents had a villa. Tracy and I had loads of freedom there because it was so safe. We'd disappear in the morning, play on the beach and when we were hungry or thirsty we'd go into cafés and bars on our own. They let us have a 'slate' so that we could order drinks and snacks on tick and later on, when the owner saw Dad, they'd tell him what he owed. It was blissful, and a good way of teaching us independence.

This confidence stood me in good stead at school. I don't recall getting bullied or picked on because I would always stand up for myself, and for anyone I loved. At one point, my cousin Helen was having a hard time at high school and I went over to the girl who was the ringleader and said: 'Don't you dare do anything to hurt my cousin, Helen! It's horrible and I love her, so you stop it now!' I had to crane my neck just to look at this girl, who was about twice my size, but I'd do anything for people who are close to me.

My parents have always been totally behind me and I couldn't imagine anything else. They taught me how to act when I met new people, how to be polite, and all the little things such as what cutlery to use at a meal – but I think Paul's upbringing had focused on different values. At any rate, he seemed totally fazed by the prospect of dinner at my family home.

Mum and Dad didn't know much about Paul before I announced that he was my boyfriend but during the following week they found out more. In fact, I felt as if I had to get both them *and* Paul ready for the big day! He was so worried about them, and they wanted to know so much about him, that I was constantly being questioned by someone or other. I was the only one who wasn't worried, because I felt sure they would get on.

My dad came out with some typical 'dad stuff' as the week went on. The morning after Paul first picked Nicky and me up to give us a lift into town the previous March, I had mentioned to Dad that he smoked, and he brought it up now. He said, 'He's 18 and he smokes, our Lindsey. You'll never be happy!' It was true I hated smoking with a passion and had always said I'd never get involved with someone who had a cigarette in their hand, but with Paul it didn't matter, and I regretted I'd mentioned it to Dad.

I couldn't really tell them about any of the problems with Gemma. Open and friendly as they were, they would have found it difficult to understand that complication. As it was, they only knew of Paul as my best friend's cousin and the lad from the estate who was doing so well at snooker.

I knew more. I knew that there was just something about him. He was the first bad lad, the first naughty lad I'd ever been drawn to. I never quite knew where I was with him and

I liked that. I told myself, 'You've taken your eye off the ball here, Lindsey Fell. What are you thinking about, falling for this one?' It didn't matter – I really liked him, and I knew my parents would too.

Sunday arrived, and I was probably the most relaxed out of everyone. Tracy had gone out with her boyfriend, Chris, and I helped Mum to get everything ready. There was enough food to feed an army, never mind one skinny 18-year-old. As I looked at the table collapsing under dishes and cutlery and glasses, for a fleeting moment I did wonder whether Paul had been right to be worried. The Queen could have come round that day and we wouldn't have been shown up.

I went round to Paul's house to pick him up and when I got there, his mum ushered me into their living room. 'Come in, Lindsey,' said Kris. 'Make yourself at home. Paul tells me he's coming for a lovely meal to your house today.' I couldn't imagine that Paul had used the word 'lovely' to describe it, but I nodded and we chatted for a bit, mostly about the holiday and work, until Paul appeared. He wore a smart shirt and trousers and had about half a ton of gel on his hair. He said goodbye to his mum, who saw us to the door quite formally, and as soon as he was in my car, he gave a huge sigh.

'I'm a wreck,' he said. 'All I'm trying to do is get you to sleep with me – it better be worth the bother,' he joked.

When we got back to my house there was no need for introductions as Paul had met my parents before, and thankfully he kept his 'Big Bad G' comments to himself. I saw his face fall as we went through to the room with the table all neatly set, but then he cheered up straight away when my dad asked him what he would like to drink.

'I'll have a vodka, please, Graham, a very large one,' Paul said. 'And if you could just keep them coming at a steady rate for the rest of the day, I'd be much obliged.' He winked and Dad laughed and somehow the ice was broken. Paul could put anyone at ease, and the tone was immediately set for the rest of the day. He was so charming that my mum and dad thought he was great from that moment on.

The food was delicious and I filled Paul's plate for him as I knew he was worried about spilling anything. As I passed it to him, I laid his fork and knife on top, and he winked at me. We had a secret little smile between us, and I felt really happy. The rest of the day was good fun – Paul relaxed once he had drunk enough, and Mum and Dad seemed tickled to have a boyfriend of mine be so engaging and entertaining. About 5pm, we had to get going as Mum and Dad had some do on at their golf club. As we stood at the door, saying goodbyes, Paul gave my mum a big kiss and said, 'Lovely meal, Pauline. I trust you'll keep to the same standards in the future when I'm round.' She giggled a bit – my mum giggled! – and he shook my dad's hand. It was perfect, it had all gone so well.

We got into my car but didn't drive for long. I parked just round the corner and leaned over to give him a huge hug. 'That wasn't so bad, was it?' I asked him. 'No, not really – but I'm a bag of nerves, Linz. I'm glad I won't have to meet them for the first time ever again. I couldn't cope.' I had to laugh – this was a professional snooker player whose job required him to stay calm while hundreds and thousands of people watched him, and he'd been scared of my family! When I dropped him off at his house, I felt so pleased. I knew his mum would be wanting a blow-by-blow account of what had happened, then he was going out with his cousin Anthony for a night out to get over his fraught day.

When I got back, Mum said, 'I don't know anything about snooker, our Lindsey, but what a nice lad he is! Your dad's heard of him, but I've no idea. Is he definitely your boyfriend now?' I said that he was, and the words sounded funny even to me. 'Well,' my mum replied, 'I don't know what you're doing with a lad so young, what with you being so sensible and so mature, but he's lovely.'

My dad agreed. 'He's just a regular nice guy; you'd never think he's got money or status. But you know what he is, Lindsey? He's a bit of a "Jack the lad".'

There was something about Paul – even my parents could see it. It had been complicated while he was on and off with Gemma, but I felt that we were on the right path now.

Over the next few weeks, things continued to go well. Paul came to our house frequently, and it soon became as natural for him to be there – and eat his dinner there – as it was at his own home. By September, my parents had accepted him totally. He was one of the family only six months after we met.

For me, the time had come. I decided to sleep with Paul for the first time. We were going out with Nicky and her new boyfriend Nobby, and then planned to go back to Paul's house to stay. Kris and Alan were away for the night and I knew that I was going to have to share a bed with Paul. I guess he realized that it might be the big night but we didn't really talk about it beforehand. I did want to sleep with him, but I was a bit worried. My only other sexual experiences had been with Dave and I was so used to him that I didn't know what to expect with another boy.

I was nervous and worried about it the whole night while we were at a club. I had a fair bit to drink but I didn't want to be so drunk that I wouldn't know what was happening. When we got back, I looked at Paul's bedroom as if I was seeing it for the first time. I'd been in there before, as we all used to hang out there when we were round at Paul's house, but this time was different. This time it was just us.

The double bed had a bold patterned duvet on it, and had been neatly made up – did his mum do that, I wondered? Would I be expected to make it again in the morning? Would I still be there in the morning?

I nervously sat on the edge of the bed while Paul cleaned his teeth. I wanted him to come in quickly and make a big joke about it. I wanted it to be over quickly so that we could relax, so that *I* could relax. But it was a different Paul who came back from the bathroom. He walked over to me, sat down on the bed and took my hand. He brushed my hair out of my face and tucked it behind my ear. There weren't any jokes. This mattered. To both of us.

He kissed me and I felt myself get tense. He must have felt it too, because he asked, 'Are you all right, Linz?' I answered quickly, 'Yeah, fine, absolutely fine.' Paul moved away from me a little and took my face in his hands. 'I can't believe you've made me wait six months for this,' he said, 'but if it's not what you want, I'll wait longer. You have to be ready, babes. You have to be sure.'

He was so tender with me that all of the worry just left my body. The next moments were private, memories that we made together that I want to keep for me. But it was quite a shock when I realized something else had happened that night, something more than just having sex with him.

I'd fallen in love with Paul Hunter.

Chapter Eight

Which girlfriend?

For a few weeks, I was the happiest girl in the world. Paul was very attentive and we went everywhere together, announcing our relationship to the world. I thought about him the whole time and found it difficult to concentrate at work, but he seemed to be thinking about me all the time as well. We were just typical young lovers. We'd jump into bed at every opportunity and we were so compatible it seemed the most natural thing in the world. I was on a high, looking forward to all the wonderful days and nights we would share together and counting the hours until I would see him again. I looked forward to our relationship getting deeper and deeper as we got to know each other better. If I had any slight worry, it was that he wasn't looking for someone to settle down with at that stage; he wasn't even looking for a long-term girlfriend, let alone someone to marry – but he didn't know what I was like once I made up my mind about something. And once my heart had decided it loved Paul, who was I to argue?

The snooker season was starting up again and players were getting their practice in and beginning to rev up for the professional year ahead. Paul was practising in earnest and I would often pop in to The Manor to see him during my lunch break, or even in between appointments. We could meet for lunch and have a quick chat on the phone whenever we liked because he didn't have a boss leaning over his shoulder. To an outsider, he might have looked like a young waster hanging around the snooker tables all day every day, while his girlfriend slaved away. I worked long hours as a full-time beauty therapist, plus all my evening work teaching at the college and sometimes seeing private clients as well, while Paul had a flexible timetable. Of course, if anybody had stopped for more than a few seconds, they would soon have realized that he was a lot more than that – his talent was incredible, even to a non-snooker aficionado like me.

However, I wasn't the only person who was hanging around Paul. One day in October, when Paul and I had been together properly for about four weeks, I walked into The Manor to see Gemma sitting in the café having a coffee. My heart gave a bit of a jolt but I told myself it was nothing. When I said to Paul, casually, 'Oh, I just saw Gemma outside,' he didn't seem to bat an eyelid. 'Did you say hello?' he asked. 'I don't think she saw me,' I replied, and told myself to forget all about it.

The following week, though, I saw her talking to Paul just outside the room where the snooker tables were. She saw me coming and walked off before I could say anything. 'What was that about?' I asked Paul. He seemed a bit flustered but maintained that she was just being friendly.

I didn't want to become suspicious – it's not in my nature – but I had a bad feeling about it. He and Gemma seemed to have been in an on-off relationship for so long, and I was worried that I hadn't seen the last of her.

I wasn't sure whether Gemma had a job or not – but she did seem to have plenty of time to hang around Paul. She started coming regularly for a coffee or a snack in the café at The Manor, and it seemed she always managed to chat to him on the way there and back. Sometimes she'd catch sight of me coming and she'd leave; other times we might exchange a polite 'hello' but it never went any further than that. I never had a conversation with Gemma at any point over the years, and I certainly didn't intend to have a public fight with her. Paul maintained it was just that they wanted to stay friends, having been together for such a long time, and I found it hard to argue with that.

One night, when Nicky and I had been out for a drink, I plucked up the courage to ask her what was going on as we made our way back to her house. 'Nicky,' I said, 'did I tell you I saw Gemma recently?' 'No,' she replied. 'Where? In town?' I knew I was going to have to tell her more, but there was a part of me that was reluctant to open the whole issue up. Maybe I was subconsciously scared of what I might hear. 'Chatting to Paul at the club,' I told her. 'She's there practically every day hanging round Paul. What's going on, Nicky?'

It turned out that Nicky was just as much out of the loop

as I was. Not only was she spending a lot of time with her new boyfriend Nobby, meaning that she often wasn't at home when Paul called round, but she was also trying to avoid knowing anything so she wasn't put in an awkward position. 'Our Darren did say that Gemma had been making a play for Paul again,' she confessed, 'but I'm in a really tricky position here, Lindsey – Paul's my cousin and I love him to bits, but you're my best mate and I'd do anything for you.'

I paused and took stock of what she had just said. 'Are you saying that you suspected something was going on, Nicky? Because if you did, I'd have thought you would have told me.' She took my hand and looked at me with those big, open eyes of hers. 'It's not like that, Linz. It's not about you. It's Paul. He's never, ever been faithful to any girl before – it just doesn't seem to be something he's capable of. There's no malice in him; he just can't help himself. And, although I don't know anything, it's just his past record that bothers me.' This was sounding worse and worse. 'Nicky,' I said, 'you've got to find out what's going on. I won't be messed about again. I need to know.'

I couldn't settle after that, and eventually got a taxi home rather than stay over. Nicky called me the next morning. 'Lindsey, I've raked our Darren over the coals about this and it's not good news, babes. Paul's back with Gemma again.'

I thanked her for letting me know and put the phone down. I didn't want to discuss this with anyone; I just wanted to work it out myself. It was only a month since we'd started sleeping together. I felt like a complete idiot for falling for his charms and jumping into bed with him. Now he had thrown everything back in my face. I'd told him how much of a big deal it was for me to have sex with him; he knew that meeting my parents properly was important to me. Did none of that matter to him? Didn't I matter to him? I went to my bedroom and had a good cry – from shock, surprise, fury, hurt and real, bitter sadness at having to let go of my beautiful dreams for our future. Once I'd cried it all out, I went into practical mode and tried to work out what was behind it all.

It was as if Paul couldn't get Gemma out of his system. They were one of those couples who seem to be attached by a piece of elastic, pinging back and forwards to each other, breaking up and making up. Perhaps it was the drama that made it addictive.

I had to take a stand, though; nobody gets to have two girlfriends, especially if one of them is me! I called him but he didn't take the call. I assumed that after Nicky had quizzed Darren, he had warned Paul that I knew. I left a message on his phone saying to call me, and that I didn't intend to keep phoning him all day. I told him I knew what was going on and I wanted a word. It was a couple of hours before he called back. Paul always hated confrontation and avoided it whenever possible, but this time he had no choice.

'Lindsey,' he said straight away, 'I know how this probably looks to you, but hear me out. You've only heard this from Nicky who heard it from Darren – give me a chance to say my piece. Please?'

'Absolutely, Paul,' I answered. 'You go for it, babes. You tell me how, when Darren told Nicky that you were with

Gemma again, that he got it all wrong. Did Darren mishear it? Did Nicky not understand what he was saying? Have you not been phoning Gemma, not seeing her, not sleeping with her again?' Of course, I didn't know for sure they were having sex again, but I assumed they were.

'Oh, Lindsey,' he pleaded. 'You make it sound so bad, but it wasn't deliberate. She just kept hanging around me.'

'And that was it? You just had to give in because she was pestering you? That, Paul Hunter, is a pathetic excuse for being unfaithful to me but it doesn't matter anyway. We're finished,' I told him.

'Now, babes,' he said, 'I know you don't mean that. I'm really sorry, really sorry. I'll finish with Gemma then we'll be fine.' His voice faltered. He knew I wasn't going to take this well.

I couldn't believe what I was hearing! 'You'll finish with her?' I said. 'You'll finish with her? For how long, Paul? A day? A week? You've "finished" with her so many times, and gone back to her so many times, that I don't think you even understand what the word means. Let me show you how it's done. We, you and me, Lindsey and Paul, are finished. Now watch and see how it really works.' With that, I put the phone down and switched it off for the rest of the day.

That evening I went round to Nicky's and her family were all really supportive. Nicky's mum – who was Paul's auntie, after all – even went so far as to say that she thought Paul was making a huge mistake, and they all thought I was perfect for him. It was ironic; everyone seemed to think that but Paul.

Funnily enough, I soon got over my initial anger with him. I know he'd cheated on me, but it wasn't about me. He had a self-destructive streak that sometimes made him spoil the things he cared about the most. In many ways he was just so young and immature, but there was still something about him that made him loveable. He was like a naughty puppy stealing a biscuit from the coffee table; you can't stay mad at them for long because they're just doing what's in their nature. However, I was determined not to back down. I wasn't a masochist, after all.

Over the following days and weeks, it got harder for me rather than easier. The problem was that I was so close to his cousin Nicky and sister Leanne that I couldn't avoid hearing about Paul, and it pickled my brain. I always knew what was happening with him and Gemma and I didn't want to know. I just needed to get over him but I didn't get the chance. Sometimes I would see them in the distance when we came out of different clubs at the same time, or I would hear from someone that they had been spotted somewhere. I'm not a jealous person but it was really painful seeing Paul with his arm round her and imagining him going home to bed with her. I tried not to torture myself with images of them together but at weak moments I couldn't help it.

And Paul? He tried to phone me a few times but I never took his calls. There was nothing to say. He'd had his chance to prove that I meant something to him and he'd treated me as though I was little more than a fling.

In the weeks after we split up, two things happened to Paul – he turned 19 and he won the Regal Welsh Open, a tournament that was being televised. He beat lots of well-known players like Steve Davis, and he even beat John Higgins in the final. I watched it at my parents' house and felt very distant from the person on the screen. The commentator said that Paul was the third youngest winner of a major professional snooker tournament of all time, after Ronnie O'Sullivan and Stephen Hendry. He was on the road to fame now, I thought. There were camera flashbulbs going off everywhere and people clapping him forever. At the end of the presentation, he was interviewed and he got the microphone and said, 'I'd really like to thank everyone for supporting me, especially my girlfriend back in Leeds.'

I nearly jumped off the sofa, my heart in my mouth! Could he possibly mean me, or was he talking about Gemma? My dad asked, 'Is he talking about you?' because I hadn't told my parents the whole story about what was going on. At that moment, I had to admit to myself that I was still in love with him. Paul had got to me; I'd loved him before, and I still loved him. The fact that he had cheated on me meant that I knew I could never trust him around Gemma again, but I still clung to the hope that he would grow up a bit and figure out what was in his best interests. Me.

Paul was in the papers a lot after he won that tournament. He'd got prize money of £60,000 and found that he had a lot of new friends hanging around, wanting to share his good fortune. He was something of a local hero in Leeds and I saw his face smiling out at me practically every time I walked past a newsstand. One night in November 1997 when I was out on the town with friends, we saw each other in a club and I managed to say 'hello', which was very hard. Most of the time he wasn't around because he was away playing, but I began to hear rumours that he was going off the rails a bit, drinking lots and not practising enough.

Meanwhile, I pulled myself together and decided to try and move on with the rest of my life. I'd always fancied buying a house of my own and this seemed like a good time, so I started viewing properties. In the back of my mind, I admit that even in this I was daydreaming that if Paul and I did get back together, we'd have somewhere we could be alone. Immediately after we split up I'd been so hurt that I was determined never to get back with him, but over time it was almost as if I had forgotten how bad it had been. I know it's crazy but I just couldn't get over him.

That Christmas, I needed some sort of project in my life to stop me from missing him, so when I saw a house I liked I moved fast. By February I had moved in. Mum and Dad helped me with the deposit and I still had my savings to buy furniture and do the place up. I started to teach full-time, while treating private clients in the evenings. The wages were good, and I felt quite steady.

From time to time I would ask Nicky and Leanne if Paul was still with Gemma. Half of the time they didn't know; they would only be able to work it out if she had been round recently. I had spent the last few months trying to get him out of my head and it had only had the opposite effect. I felt as though I was thinking about him all the time. I should have known that I wouldn't be able to get him out of my system so quickly. He'd got a hold on me in the first place without me having any say in it, and now he was under my skin. Turned out I wasn't as sensible as I'd always thought – I was certainly a complete fool for Paul Hunter.

Chapter Nine

The lost years

1998–2000

By the spring of 1998, I'd settled into my own house and was feeling really confident about life in general. I was still running between three different jobs, but it was worth it. I managed to fit in a good social life and had lots of friends. My parents and my sister Tracy came round to visit me all the time and I felt as if everything had fallen into place.

Apart from Paul.

My friend Vicky had moved into the house with me, and she was going through a really bad time; the lad she had been with for 10 years had split up with her and she was in shock because she'd thought they would be together forever. We were like two Bridget Joneses. We'd stay in at the weekend with a bottle of wine moaning about men. Vicky would say, 'When are we going to meet lads we really like?' I'd say, 'Well, I've found mine but he doesn't want me!'

I used to talk about Paul all the time. I must have driven my friends up the wall, because they would often tell me to get over him and find somebody else – and shut up about it. If I was a friend of mine, I'd have been saying the same thing. The pain was constant – it was as if being away from him physically and emotionally for those months had made me want him even more. I was pining for Paul.

Paul had treated me so badly but I still really liked him. How many thousands of girls out there will be able to sympathize with that? Something happens when you fall in love, especially when it's seemingly one-sided. You don't even recognize yourself any more. I knew that, if I wanted him, I'd either have to stick it out until he grew up or try to change him somehow. But how?

One night in March, I went into town on a Saturday night with Nicky and some other girls, and we saw Paul a few tables down from us in a club. Nicky said to me, 'Look at him, Lindsey. He's out with his friends, meant to be having a good time, but he just looks really unhappy.' I could see what she was getting at – he was acting as if everything was great, buying drinks for everybody and laughing, but every so often he would just look miserable, especially when he was left on his own if the others were away getting drinks or having a dance. I knew that I was being soft but I decided to go up and speak to him.

'All right, Paul,' I said. 'Lindsey!' he exclaimed, turning round in his chair to see me. 'I noticed you were over there with Nicky but I didn't know if you'd want me to come over.' I felt sorry for him – we had to get this sorted; even if we weren't going to be together, I knew that I still wanted to be friends with him. 'No Gemma tonight, Paul?' I asked him.

'No Gemma for a lot of nights,' he said quietly. 'We've had a fight.' I just nodded.

'Look, Paul, I think we need to get a few things sorted.'

'Are you going to shout at me, Lindsey?' he asked, and we both smiled, knowing that shouting wasn't quite my style. 'No,' I said. 'But Paul – you hurt me, you really did. I trusted you and you threw that back in my face. You lied to me and you cheated on me. I don't ever want that to happen to me again, whether it's by you or someone else.'

He interrupted me. 'I know, Linz, and I'm so, so, so sorry. If I could go back and change things I would. It's just that Gemma and I have been together such a long time. It's hard to walk away. I'm confused. I don't know what to do.'

Paul and I chatted a bit more and had a dance together. One of the girls I was with had tickets for another club so we all left before him and his mates.

Years later, when Paul and I were together properly, I asked him what had really been going on in that period. He said that he knew he loved me – but thought what he felt for Gemma was love too, and just couldn't decide. Because they'd been so young when they got together, she had a hold over him, whereas I intrigued him. I had my own car, my own house, a good job; I didn't need his money, and he didn't know what to do with me. Perhaps something in him liked her dependence on him, whereas he could see that I was my own person. If they fell out, he'd have to take her home; I'd just say, 'Bye, Paul!' and drive off.

At the time, knowing that Paul was torn between us was enough to make me think that I should give him another chance. Maybe if I stayed strong and supportive, he would be able to make a final break from her. If I could just hang in there, I knew he was worth it.

A few weeks after Paul and I talked in the club, he called me and asked if I would like to go for a meal. He sounded quite upset so I agreed and he picked me up from work that night. We went to a restaurant nearby and he started pouring his heart out to me almost straight away.

'Lindsey, things aren't going too well,' he said. I knew that he wasn't just referring to the situation with Gemma. Nicky had told me that Paul's snooker was going from bad to worse. He was drinking too much, smoking too much marijuana, and practising too little. His ranking had gone down and he was in real danger of becoming a wasted talent. It was as if he thought he didn't need to do any hard work, and he drank vodka into oblivion. That night he told me all of this in his own words, and I listened as if it was news to me.

When he was finished, I said, 'Paul, it's fine to do all of that stuff off season, but not when you are meant to be working. Snooker is your job and you don't seem to be applying yourself so it's only natural that things have got worse.' I don't know if anyone had ever given it straight to Paul like that but to me, it was the same as if he had been working in an office or a factory. 'You should do your job properly and don't go looking for sympathy if you are the one mucking things up for yourself.'

'God, Linz,' he said, once I had finished my speech. 'You don't beat around the bush, do you?'

'There's no point, Paul. If you choose to throw everything away, you have to realize that you are the one to blame. You could have the world at your feet if you wanted it.'

'And would you be there beside me, Lindsey?' he asked, taking my hand.

I fell for it all. Of course I did.

That night was lovely. We finished our meal and then went back to my house. It was the first time Paul had been there. 'You're quite the property tycoon, aren't you?' he joked as he walked in. 'Maybe you'll be the one keeping me in luxury.' I made some coffee, but we both knew what was going to happen next. As we sat on the sofa, Paul put his arm around me and drew me towards him. 'I've missed you so much,' he whispered in my ear. 'Enough to stop seeing Gemma?' I asked. 'Anything,' he answered. 'Anything.'

I knew I was being a fool to myself, but as we kissed and made our way to the bedroom, I had to believe what he was saying. I didn't want to be without him any longer, and I did think we had made some progress that night. He had confided in me his worries about his snooker and I had shown that he could always trust me to tell him the truth. I thought that sort of honesty was just the type of thing you built relationships on, and a relationship with Paul was exactly what I wanted. I really thought this was a new beginning.

I hoped I had got through to him, but when he left in the morning, I felt a knot of dread in my stomach. Was he going to *her* now? He called me that afternoon to say he had really enjoyed our time together and hoped we could do it again next weekend. I was starry-eyed and said 'yes', but when I went round to Nicky's a few nights later to tell her about Paul and me getting back together, she told me something before I could even start. 'Sorry, I couldn't phone you last night,' she said. 'Paul was here on the bloody thing for hours – our bill's about trebled because of him and Gemma.'

'He was calling Gemma?' I asked, my heart sinking into my boots.

'Isn't he always?' Nicky replied.

I decided not to tell Nicky I'd been seeing him again as I knew she would have divided loyalties. Instead, I called Paul as soon as I got home that night. 'Paul,' I began, 'I need to know something – are we together or not?' He didn't even try to lie; he just groaned. 'Oh, Linz, I know what this is about. I didn't mean to mess you about, it's just that … I just can't … oh, this is a mess, isn't it?'

It turned out that the night we spent together was the start of the whole cycle repeating itself and I should have guessed it. It went on for months and months on end; in fact, all through 1998 and right into the following year. I'd bump into Paul, we'd get chatting, then I'd sleep with him and think we were together again, only to hear that he was back with Gemma. I hated myself for it, but it was as if I was addicted – I also knew, in my heart of hearts, that he was the one for me.

I'd heard that his snooker was still going downhill and that he hadn't paid a blind bit of attention to my advice. He was spending far too much time partying and far too little time practising. He was in nightclubs more than snooker clubs, and he always seemed to be in the newspapers for the wrong reasons. I thought that maybe I could be the one to save him from himself, if only I got the chance – he needed someone to look out for him – but he would have to make the decision to be with me and only me first.

Before I had met him, back in 1996 he had gone to a snooker tournament in Blackpool and was mucking about on the promenade late one night with Matthew Stevens, a very close snooker player friend. Matthew and Paul had made their way through snooker qualifying school together and they were two young lads who liked to have a beer and muck around. That night in Blackpool, they both decided to have a bit of a laugh, and started taking their clothes off. Paul only got down to his t-shirt and boxers (he was always a bit self-conscious about being so skinny), but Matthew went the whole hog and streaked along Blackpool pier. They both got their clothes back on and were fully dressed by the time the police car appeared. Someone had reported that there was a naked man wandering through Blackpool and they were there to make sure someone was reprimanded. It was reported in all the papers that Paul Hunter had been fined for streaking, but no one ever got the real story. Paul knew that Matthew's family would be horrified if their son was caught stripping in public, even if it was only two drunk lads having a laugh. So, when the police arrived and asked who had been starkers, Paul took the blame. He was already developing a naughty, bad boy image, so he reasoned it was easier for him to take the rap – even though it resulted in him being disciplined and fined by the World Professional Billiards and Snooker Association for his behaviour. This was one of the earliest of the 'bad boy' stories to reach the press, but it set a pattern and there would be lots more to come.

The months went on and I struggled to cope with the Paul and Gemma situation. I had never been messed around like that in my life. I wouldn't do it to somebody and I wouldn't have expected to have it done to me but I was completely under Paul Hunter's spell. Each time, after he'd hurt me, he would be contrite and sad and confused and desperate to make up again. He seemed to be getting hooked on me as well, but at the same time he couldn't let go of Gemma.

I didn't recognize myself; I couldn't get away no matter how hard I tried. Whenever I phoned his sister or Nicky for a natter, I'd ask, 'Is she there?' If they said that she was, I felt as if my heart was being ripped out.

I decided I would try to meet somebody else. For about six months I tried to play Paul at his own game. I met and dated four different lads, trying to find someone to help me get over Paul, but it just wasn't working. I went out with one of them, a lad called Chris, for about two months. He was six foot four, had a good job, was well dressed and I did like him – but at the back of my mind I was thinking about how jealous Paul would feel when he saw me out in town with Chris. It worked to an extent. Paul started calling me a lot more while I was seeing Chris.

I was driving another lad home to Wakefield one night

and it was announced on the radio that Paul Hunter was in a local tournament. I looked across at this poor boy and thought, 'What am I doing with you?' Even when I went for a cheekier sort, they didn't appeal the way Paul did. Instead of finding someone to take my mind off him, I kept thinking that there was something he had that they didn't. I kept trying to get away then I kept going back to him.

I could never be cross with Paul for long because I knew he wasn't being deliberately malicious or nasty. He was just torn. He would say that he was the one who was suffering because he loved us both. What a nerve – trying to get sympathy from me when he was sleeping with someone else!

One night I was at home expecting Paul to come over. As I sat there in my red pyjamas, I just knew he was up to something. My friend Karen was there and she said, 'You two are meant to be together. I can see you married.' I replied, 'Well, maybe, but in the meantime he'll have me institutionalized; I'm going doolally here.'

I phoned him but his mobile was switched off. He would only do that for one reason – because he was with Gemma. When he was out with me, he would switch the mobile off so that Gemma couldn't reach him. She must have been going through the same experiences as me, feeling just as upset about it all yet unable to break away and move on.

I hated feeling out of control, so I decided I would catch him out and let him *know* that I had caught him out. We got in the car, both of us in pyjamas, and drove to Gemma's house. I pulled up opposite and there was Paul's car in the drive. I got such a burst of rage that I wanted to let his tyres down; I wanted to knock on Gemma's door and drag them out of bed. I couldn't be that nasty, though. Instead, I wrote a note to leave on his windscreen saying that I knew he was there – but then I decided not to leave it. I thought I'd wait and see whether he lied to me when I next spoke to him.

The next day he was full of life and chatting away. He started to tell me about this club he'd been to, what road he'd taken to get there, how the battery on his mobile was flat. I suddenly broke in. 'Why are you lying to me, Paul?' He was defensive straight away. 'What do you mean? I'm not lying. Why do you think I'm lying?' I told him I had been to Gemma's house and seen his car in her drive. 'Are you a stalker, Lindsey?' he asked with a straight face. 'You're supposed to be sorry, Paul,' I said. 'You're supposed to be begging my forgiveness.' He looked at me and said 'Right,' and just smiled that cheeky grin of his. 'That's it then!' I shouted. 'We're done. We're finished for good now.' He whisked me up in his arms, and carried me through to the bedroom, laughing and saying, 'Fair enough, we're over – let's just do this first though!'

He was so cheeky, always laughing, that he made me act against my better judgement every time. When he ended up back with Gemma, each time I thought to myself it was the last straw but we always ended up back together again, back in bed, back in each other's arms.

I knew that I would have to do something to break the cycle I was stuck in. It wasn't that I didn't love Paul – far from it – I just thought I wasn't being true to myself. I decided to change my job and get away from Leeds, so I found a vacancy working for Virgin as a therapist on long-haul flights. I filled in all the application forms and was invited to an interview in London. In my mind, I decided: 'If I get this job, I'm not meant to be with Paul. If I don't and I stay in Leeds, I'll do everything in my power to get him.' Everything centred around Paul; my parents and Tracy had no idea of what I was going through. I didn't want them to hate him just in case we ever did get together properly so I never told them about Gemma.

As it happened I didn't get the job, and I convinced myself that it was fate. Meanwhile, some of the students at the college where I taught told me they wanted to do a course called Beauty Therapy, NVQ Level 3, but our college didn't offer it. I approached my old college where I had trained and told them; they were keen but had no one to teach it so they offered me a job setting up a new course. It was a private college within The Manor – the very health club where Paul practised every day. I thought it was destiny. From then on, every day I'd walk past his snooker table and, if we'd had a fall out, he'd say 'Hiya Linz', and we'd eventually fall back into seeing each other again.

When we were on, it was lovely. I'd meet him for lunch and see him throughout the day and then he'd come back with me at night to my house. But he might do that for a couple of weeks and then it would all go wrong. It wasn't just that he was always seeing other girls; he also went to casinos, stayed out late, and had nights out with the boys. Paul was just, as my dad had said, Jack the lad. That was the snooker lifestyle. In summer 1999, he was still being a bit of a waster. He didn't live near any of the other professional snooker players so the guys he'd hang out with when he was off season were just bums. They didn't have jobs and they just sponged off Paul. He had to sort his life out.

Paul's twenty-first birthday, in October 1999, fell right in the middle of the snooker Grand Prix in Bournemouth. I knew he would be getting mashed on the night of his birthday, but I didn't realize quite how self-destructive he was capable of being. The next day, he was one of the players randomly selected for a drugs test – and his was positive. The press reported it as a birthday prank gone wrong – that Paul had 'stupidly tried a joint' – but everyone around him knew that it was evidence that he just didn't think further ahead than the moment he was in. It was no way for a professional sportsman to behave and the governing body agreed. They decreed that Paul would have to forfeit his prize money for reaching the last 16 of the competition as well as having some of his ranking points docked. And he did. He took his punishment without a word of complaint – and, in many ways, it did him the world of good.

When he got back, I gave him a few home truths about how he was throwing everything away and for once he didn't laugh. 'I know you're right, Lindsey,' he admitted. 'This is all I've ever wanted to do – snooker is all that I *can* do. I don't want to lose everything, Linz, I don't want that to happen.' I gave him a cuddle and told him that I'd always be there for him. It was a big thing for me to say because it was almost tantamount to admitting that he could mess me around as much as he liked, but I did feel we were turning a corner now; what had happened to him, the points docking and forfeiting his prize money, may have given him the wake-up call he needed.

I don't look back on those years as wasted. Now that our time together has been cut short, I suppose I could feel bitter about it. I could feel that we missed out on extra years when we could have been together – but he just wasn't ready for a steady relationship back then. It was part of who he was; he needed to sow his wild oats to get them out of his system. Given what he was going to be facing later, I'm almost glad he did.

When was the beginning of our love? Maybe we were always right for each other and there wasn't a specific start to it; we just had to meet, get over those early tricky times, then stick together come hell or high water. I'd made my decision. For better or worse, I was going to stick by him now.

Chapter Ten

Polishing the diamond
2000–2001

N icky, Leanne and I were sitting having a coffee one day when talk turned to Paul, as it often did. All three of us round that table loved him dearly, but it was becoming clear, even to us, that he was sabotaging his own future. Paul's wild days had to stop. For the past year or so he had been drunk or stoned pretty much all of the time; and this, in turn, had interfered with his professional life resulting in a drop in his ranking. In fact, some people were writing him off as a flash in the pan, either a gifted childhood player who had thrown it all away, or someone who had only had temporary brilliance and hadn't been able to hack it as a professional adult competitor on the circuit.

Paul's dad, Alan, was still acting as his manager, just as he had done since Paul was a little boy. He arranged contracts, sponsors and matches and accompanied him to tournaments. I often wondered how Alan managed to separate being Paul's father from being his manager. One thing was becoming obvious though – it wasn't working. Alan didn't

UnbreakableUnbreakable

seem to have the authority to keep Paul off the drugs and booze. Paul did as he pleased and Alan couldn't get him under control, any more than I could. If Alan said 'black', Paul would do 'white' and there was nothing he could do about it.

Around this time, Paul was attracting attention on the snooker circuit and an agent and manager called Brandon Parker came along who would become his professional saviour and a great friend as well. Brandon was well respected on the circuit and had taken an immediate liking to Paul when they had met the previous year. He had been watching Paul for a while, and was well aware of his talent. At the time, Brandon was representing a player called Mark Miller and had invested £10,000 in him to see if he was good enough to make the grade. Brandon decided to set up a matches between Paul and Mark Miller – and Paul buried him. It was enough to make the well-respected manager start watching the golden-haired lad even more closely.

Brandon had also managed an Australian player called Quinten Hann and he recognized that there were changes happening in the snooker world. For the guys at the top, image was becoming as important as talent. Following Brandon's advice, Quinten had his hair dyed, changed the colour of his waistcoat, and made a few other little cosmetic changes and they resulted in him getting a lot more newspaper coverage. Quinten felt more confident going into matches and Brandon had guided him from a ranking of 106 all the way to number 14 in the world. Obviously this was much more to do with talent than waistcoat colour, but it showed that Brandon really knew how to put a package together. Snooker had been so popular in the 1980s and had had huge characters like Alex Higgins, but it had become dull in the 1990s and many people felt it was time for a renaissance. If there was any chance of someone bringing a bit of life to the sport, he would be welcomed.

Paul could beat Quinten fairly easily and that convinced Brandon that he wanted to manage him and could do a lot with him. Personally I was delighted when Brandon Parker arrived on the scene. It was clear that Paul needed some professional input and this guy really seemed to know what he was doing.

I suppose it was telling that, one day in early 2000, Paul asked me to go with him to meet Brandon. He hadn't asked Gemma, and I knew that he was spending more time with me and less with her. Paul told me that he liked this guy and wanted to work with him, but seemingly Brandon had asked to meet me too.

Brandon drove over from his home in Manchester and the three of us met for coffee and a chat at my house. Paul introduced me as his girlfriend.

'Lindsey,' said Brandon once we had all sat down, 'I won't mince my words – I've told Paul already that he's been having it easy. When he wins, he finds it smooth going because he doesn't even bother to practise. Fair enough – but he's not winning enough. When you lose that thread, it's hard to get it back, but I can help him. I want to help him. You've maybe won a few things, Paul, but from what I can see, you've had 18 months of struggling. Your sponsorship contracts could be negotiated better as well – some of them aren't doing you any favours.'

Brandon was right but it had been hard for Paul not to feel guilty about the prospect of taking on a new manager when his father had been looking after him up to that point. That's one of the problems when you work with family. Besides, Paul usually paid very little attention to the contractual and financial side of things. He nodded throughout Brandon's speech but didn't really say anything, so it was up to me to add my bit.

'I'm sure you're completely straight, Brandon,' I told him, 'but it's easy to say that contracts are rubbish when what you really want is to get Paul on your team. You're not doing this out of the kindness of your heart – what are you offering?'

Brandon grinned. 'You've got a good one there, Paul,' he said, and I could see Paul shine with pride. 'I'll tell you exactly what I'm offering, Lindsey – nothing,' he said, to our surprise. 'You need to trust me on your terms, Paul, so let's try this tack. I won't ask you to sign a binding contract for a year until you've seen what I can do for you. How does that sound?'

'It sounds like an offer you can't refuse, babes,' I said to Paul as I squeezed his hand. There was still something bothering him though. 'My dad?' he asked Brandon. 'What happens with my dad?'

'Don't you worry about any of that,' said Paul's new manager. 'Your dad will still be involved. We'll meet him next week to get things sorted out. Paul, I think you are an absolutely unbelievable player and you have a totally unique character. From what I've seen, you've got the ability to get on with everyone – but you also have the ability to be the best at this game. My job is to take the pressure off, and you need that. You just pot balls and I'll do everything else.'

We all shook hands. Paul went to the loo and Brandon took the opportunity to have a few words with me on my own. 'I had to meet you, Lindsey. I always have to see what the girlfriends are like. If it turned out that you were just some daft kid who wanted to blow his money, I had to know. That isn't what I've got here today at all,' he said, smiling. 'I can work with you; together we'll make this boy a star.'

After Brandon left that day, Paul and I had a spring in our step. He seemed perfect. The following week Brandon sat down with father and son and made the deal that would stand Paul in such good stead – both professionally and personally, as Brandon would soon become one of our closest friends.

After the deal was agreed, Paul popped round to my house to let me know how things had gone, and we had a glass of wine while he recounted the day.

'Linz,' he said, 'I've been thinking about things for the past few weeks. I know that I've got to get myself sorted. All I want is to play snooker and I honestly think I can get back on track with that.'

'Of course you can, babes. You've got the talent; you just need to put the hard work in too,' I told him.

'I know, I know – but there's something else, Lindsey. I don't want to do it on my own, I want to do it with you by my side. God knows what I've been thinking, but it's time to get things right for once.'

My heart was leaping, but we'd been here before and I wasn't going to push Paul. 'Whatever you want to do is fine by me,' I told him.

'I've already done it.'

'You've done what?'

'I've finished with Gemma – and before you say that I'm not very good at that, it's different this time.'

'How?' I asked him.

'Because I've told her that I've finally had enough. I told her that you were the one for me, and she finally seemed to accept it. I think we both just realized that it's daft – we hardly even talk to each other any more and I'm always round here. I don't want to be with her ever again, Lindsey. I want you.'

I was almost crying with happiness – and so was Paul. We just sat there for ages, laughing and kissing. I felt so close to him and so pleased that he had at last realized what I had known all along – that we were made for each other. It took him more than three years from when we'd first met in March 1997 till the summer of 2000, but at last it seemed we were solid and settled.

A few weeks later Brandon invited us for lunch at his house in Manchester, where we met his wife Charlotte. They were both absolutely lovely and made us so welcome. They just chatted away during the meal, then Paul and I followed Brandon through to his office – it was time to talk about the campaign.

Brandon cut to the chase straight away. 'Drugs. Women. Booze. There's no point shying away from it, Paul. You've been daft. But you're young and it can be tempting. Make no mistake, though – this is where the hard work begins. You've already been caught with marijuana in your system after that random drugs test, you've been fined and you've lost points. I'm not asking you to be an angel, just clever. You're a lad from a council estate who has been thrown into a different world but if you want to stay in that world, it's up to you. I can tell you about windows in your schedule when you can do what you like, but you need to make sure there's nothing in your system when it comes to drug tests – marijuana stays in your blood for 21 days, son, and you'd better remember that. Summer is fine, and there's a bit of a gap at Christmas too, but you need to get more controlled, and I'll make you a structured and professional regime.'

To be honest, I was shocked by all this. I was so straight-laced that I was still having a problem with Paul smoking cigarettes, never mind anything else. Brandon had a school report type checklist for his players, aimed at helping them to improve. It covered items such as body language, media appeal and looks, break building and safety, and Paul scored highly on them all. Brandon really helped with his mental attitude more than anything. Paul was still in a slump when they started but Brandon told him that he had to work on his groundwork because the flashes of brilliance came in isolation. He said that they didn't need to work on his strengths, just his weaknesses.

He spoke to Paul about the psychology of the game in a way that no one had ever done before. He talked to him about the fact that when lads like him were out there at that table, they were completely alone in front of millions. Psychologically, Paul had to get back on form. Brandon said that when Paul came out in a break from a game, it would be vital that the people he saw would be the ones who would help him. He didn't need false promises; he didn't need anything negative; he just needing polishing.

While there were matches going on, Paul needed to practise and apply himself. Trust was a big issue for Paul – and he trusted Brandon Parker completely. I think Brandon made Paul accept that he was an adult, and that was a hard lesson for him to learn. When a lad is nine years old and playing snooker 10 hours a day, he doesn't grow up. He doesn't develop social skills; some lads stay immature well into adulthood. Paul was easily bored as well and that could get him into trouble.

Brandon came into his life like a breath of fresh air. From then on, on the dead days, when there were no matches, he would take him away to keep him fresh. They played lots of golf together. One day they went to Plymouth to view boats in the marina, and they pretended they wanted to buy one. Paul came back with all these tales of them both saying to the agent, 'No, we need something bigger! What else have you got?'

Paul adored Brandon and Charlotte, and the feeling was mutual. We started spending more and more time with them and they were nothing but a good influence. I've got a photograph of the four of us together on a night out somewhere. We're all so full of life, so happy, with everything ahead of us. It's hard to believe that the youngest one of the four of us, the one with the biggest smile, the greatest lust for life, is gone now. The three of us who are left have such holes in our days now that he is gone, but he also gave us such happiness while he was here.

I wish Brandon had been around when I first met Paul – he might have saved me some heartache. As it was, he didn't just influence Paul's public and professional sides; he affected our personal life too. I had someone in my corner and Paul would finally see what I'd been trying to tell him for years – that we were made for each other; we could be an unbeatable team.

Chapter Eleven

Plan B

2001

When the big snooker tournaments were on, there was always a lot of newspaper coverage. Paul was becoming more of a recognizable figure to the media, but they all still hankered after the glory days of the late 1970s and 1980s when there were so many big personalities around. However, with Brandon's help, Paul was being groomed to achieve the same status through a combination of his talent and his looks.

One of the biggest tournaments of the year was the Masters, which takes place at Wembley in February. In 2001, Brandon told Paul that he had a real shot at it, and that this could be his big break. I didn't go down for the early stages because I was working and couldn't take the time off. I did enjoy watching snooker, but only really when Paul was playing and if I had been there, I might have distracted him. Every day, Paul would ring me before he played his match, and I'd follow his progress in the papers and on the TV.

Paul was becoming known as a bit of a 'pressure player' in

that he didn't seem to be at all bothered when he was behind in a game. When he was losing, he would still come out with a smile on his face and bagfuls of confidence. The bright lights and big crowds didn't bother him in the slightest – in fact, he loved it all. One of his problems was that he often let things slip – he could be well ahead and then just not close the match, or he let his opponent get too far away from him at the start. A lot of the time that didn't matter as he would win anyway, but I wondered whether he enjoyed that sort of pressure. He certainly had the talent to deal with it, and the nail-biting finales to many of his games were crowd-pleasers that would raise the roof of a venue.

In the 2001 Masters at Wembley, he was falling into that pattern again. He had got through every round, but often by the skin of his teeth. Every time he called to let me know how things had gone, I'd ask him the same question first: 'Did you win?' If I didn't know how it had all turned out, I couldn't bear to hear the details of how close it had been, or how tight every frame had seemed. Only after he told me that everything was OK could I let him dissect it bit by bit. That year at Wembley, every time he called the news was fantastic – he was winning every time. During the tournament he beat his friend Matthew Stevens 6–5 in the last sixteen. Matthew was the defending champion. He then beat Peter Ebdon 6–3 in the quarter-finals and Stephen Hendry 6–4 in the semi-finals. We had both decided that if Paul got into the final, I would go to London to be there for him.

He did, and he was to play Fergal O'Brien. Brandon's wife Charlotte and I drove down with Kris and Paul's sister

Leanne. I wanted to support him, but my heart would be in my mouth the whole time. I knew how much he wanted this. He had won a title already, he was ranked number 14 in the world, but this, the Masters, was a big one. This would really send out a message to everyone about how great Paul Hunter was.

Brandon met us when we arrived as Paul was busy practising. He was excited about what Paul had achieved so far and truly believed that, if he won this, his career would take off in a way we couldn't even imagine. 'He's got everything, Lindsey,' Brandon told me. 'The talent, the looks, the personality – and you. You're part of it.'

When we got to the players' hotel, Paul was waiting for me. He was so happy that day and totally focused on what he had to do. He was called to start preparing for the final, and I went to watch it all from the players' lounge. In those days, there was always lots of free drink and people would get quite jolly while they were watching the TV screening of what was going on in the main hall. Most players' wives and families didn't go into the hall itself in case the players saw them and got distracted. It was a really nice atmosphere as I knew some of the women from going to a few games before, and everyone was very friendly. That atmosphere changed a bit for me as the interval came and Paul was losing significantly, 6–2 down.

In Masters finals, there are two sessions of snooker: the first session is eight frames and the second is 11. In between, the players are allowed to stop for two hours so that they can relax, perhaps get something to eat, practise if they feel like it, or, for most of them, get some positive game talk from their manager. By the time I saw Brandon, he had already had a word with Paul. He'd told him that he was doing well, that he could turn this round, and that we were all behind him. Paul pulled on a denim jacket and turned up the collar to disguise his dickie bow and waistcoat as he walked back to his hotel room to rest. Brandon suggested I go over to see him.

'Lindsey,' he said, 'See if you can relax him. He's trying too hard – he can win this, he just needs to believe in himself.' I said I would do what I could but, to be honest, I wasn't sure what I could add given that Brandon and Paul usually worked on this side of things themselves. 'Do what you can, love,' he said. 'Just go back to the room and say to him that we all love him no matter what. It's not a big thing if he wins or loses – if he loses this time, he'll get it next year or the year after. This is meant for him, Linz. Just chill him out, give him a back massage if he wants it, or let him sleep.'

'All right, Brandon, I'll do what I can,' I said, heading off.

On the way to the hotel room, we passed lots of Paul's fans and they knew who I was – they seem to find out every single detail of their favourite players' lives. The ones that recognized us were shouting, 'Tell him he can do it!' and 'Tell Paul we love him and he's a winner!' It felt so strange hearing them chanting behind me as I went to see if I could cheer Paul up.

He was really depressed when I got to the room. 'I'm 6–2 down, Linz,' he said, as if I wouldn't know. 'I'm fed up. I'm pissing this away and I just can't be bothered with it all.' He seemed so miserable that I didn't think of him as Paul Hunter the big snooker star; he was just my bloke and he was down in the dumps. 'Relax and have something to eat,' I told him, but he was like a kid who decides that they're in a bad mood and won't be brought out of it. 'I don't want anything to eat, I don't want anything,' he said. I shrugged my shoulders and went to run a bath. A nice hot soak with bubbles always helps me and I thought it might work for him too. 'Come on, Paul!' I shouted. 'No point in being miserable, come and have a bath.'

Once he got in, I went through to the bedroom for a lie down. I didn't know what else I could say to Paul, but I knew that I would be there for him whatever happened. When he was washed and had a towel on, he lay down beside me and I gave him a kiss and a cuddle. I said, 'What's the worst that could happen? Even if you lose, you're a Masters finalist, your ranking will go up and you'll earn a decent amount of money. That's not so bad, is it? If you lose, you lose, babes.'

Paul moved closer to me and we started to kiss some more. What happened next was only natural. He slipped my top off and started removing the rest of my clothes. 'You're right, Linz,' he said. 'You're always right. How about we try this to relax?' We had a good giggle and I said that I wondered whether this was what other players did in the intervals.

Once we had made love, Paul sat up. 'Here, Lindsey,' he laughed, 'I've got an appetite now – I'll have that food you suggested after all.' We just mucked about for the rest of the break: I had a bath, he had a sleep and then he went back to the table much happier. Something must have worked because, unbelievably, Paul went on to win 10–9, including four centuries in six frames.

Unbreakable

As the cheers went up, I rushed through from the players' lounge to congratulate him. I threw my arms around him and was so full of pride, I could have burst. I just wanted to celebrate with my wonderful, wonderful bloke. There were things to do first though – there was the presentation of the trophy, which was marvellous, and then there were the drug tests and then the press interviews, which were generally very dull. After a win, there was always a press call in one of the little rooms behind the main arena. Because it was a Sunday that day, there were several other journalists, desperate for a story to go in the Monday papers, as well as the usual sports hacks. The ones who didn't work for the sports pages were all sitting up the back of the room, bored out of their skulls, probably thinking it would be a miracle if they could get a decent story out of a snooker tournament.

Paul was buzzing with adrenaline from the match. He was carrying an old gold yachting trophy worth £60,000, together with a cheque for £190,000, and he had just won one of snooker's major tournaments.

In the press room the sports journalists started praising Paul and asking him about different shots and frames. 'You were rubbish in the first session Paul, and then tonight you have been nothing short of brilliant. What changed ?'

Another chipped in: 'What did you do in the interval that made such a difference to your game? What did you think about and how did you muster up the strength to come back? What's your secret?'

Paul was on such a high with winning that he couldn't have stopped himself from answering truthfully even if he

97

had tried. As always, he was just totally honest. 'Well,' he said, 'I went for Plan B.'

There was a hushed silence, everyone wondering what this was going to be.

He continued: 'I hadn't seen my girlfriend for a while because I've been playing here, but she came down from Leeds today. I had to do something to break the tension, so we put Plan B into action – if you know what I mean.'

It was bedlam.

The non-sports journalists rushed down from the back of the room, some of them knocking their chairs over as they pushed past each other. All the tabloids were there and they were all asking Paul questions at the same time. 'You had sex, Paul? Is that your secret? Is that what helped you to win? Where's your girlfriend?' They were all delighted because they had a story now.

I was in the VIP lounge, but someone came to get me saying that the photographers wanted pictures of both of us together. I was happy to oblige because I was feeling so proud of him. Maybe I was a little bit tipsy because I'd been having a few free drinks in the players' lounge. When the photographers started asking us for certain poses, I agreed because they said there would be a lovely picture of both of us in the Monday morning editions. It took ages – look at the camera, look this way, look away from each other, all different combinations. Someone even said, 'Lindsey! Stick your tongue in his ear, love!' and I did, for a laugh, thinking it was such a daft thing to do.

Once the press call was finally over we all celebrated

together and Paul was on one of the biggest highs of his life. 'This is it, son,' said Brandon. 'This is where your life changes.'

The next morning, we heard the thud of newspapers being thrown down outside our hotel room door. Paul scrambled out of bed to get them and brought them back to where I was still half-asleep.

He was everywhere. All the headlines were about his Masters win – and something gradually dawned on us. They weren't just at the back of the paper, on the sports pages – they were on the front pages too. They all had variations on the same headline: 'Plan B works for Hunter!' And they all had photos of us beside the articles, but the pictures they used were the ones of me sticking my tongue in Paul's ear. I thought they would be of us smiling together, pictures to be proud of. Instead I looked like some horrible, drunken hanger-on.

The stories were pretty lurid too – there was one in a tabloid that said I was half naked wearing only a black g-string and bra as I crawled on all fours across the bed. I just kept thinking, My dad's going to read this! Other stories suggested that it was all Brandon Parker's idea to get more publicity for Paul; that was really insulting, I thought. How cheap must people think I am if they believe I would have sex with my boyfriend on the orders of his manager just so we could all get in the tabloids? I'd never have someone order me to have sex with Paul and then talk about it on camera. When we made love in the hotel during the break, the last thing I was thinking about was having sex so that people would know who Paul was. It wasn't a strategy – we were just a young couple who loved each other.

All that day I kept thinking, Oh my God, my dad! oh my God my dad! oh my God. Everyone I knew would see those images and read those stories – clients, family, all my students, the parents of those students! I'd been sensible all my life up to that point and now they'd think I was an idiot.

The story ran all week in the press, with journalists quizzing other professional sportsmen about whether they indulged in sexual relief during the intervals in their matches, for example at half time in a football match. Would it improve their performance?

I had been incredibly stupid at that press call but I also learned very quickly. I would never pose for a picture again without thinking it through. Paul didn't get any media training, so he was always very naive about the press, but I became careful from that moment on. He just said what he wanted, when he wanted. He always told me that once you've said something you've said it, there's no point worrying about how it's going to be used.

Plan B certainly changed things because it became a phrase that people automatically associated with Paul Hunter. They would wink at us during tournaments and ask what we had planned for the interval. It was water off a duck's back for Paul, who probably made as many jokes as anyone else, but it bothered me to begin with as I worried about how people would perceive me. Later, when Paul told the truth – that he won the Masters because he hit the balls at the right time into the right pocket – people still preferred the Plan B story.

Whatever anyone chose to believe, it all added up to one thing – Paul Hunter was becoming a household name. Over the next two years, things would just get bigger and bigger. Plan B made Paul very attractive to magazines as well as newspapers and he was asked to do photo shoots with *FHM* and *Esquire*. He was so natural in front of the camera that these were rarely one-off features. Everybody loved Paul because not only did he have an undoubted ability to look good in photos, but once journalists met him they realized he had a genuinely appealing nature. They loved his 'bad boy' image and often included him in their 'Top 10 of naughty sports stars' and similar features. Of course, by this time Paul had calmed down and the things he was becoming famous for – the sex sessions, the kiss-and-tell stories, the drugs – were all in his past. Since he had returned fully committed to the game after his wild years, Paul had turned himself round – and that was demonstrated by how well he was doing professionally.

After every win, people would ask him about Plan B again. Actually, any time we were together and Paul had a break during games, we'd joke about it ourselves. Paul would say, 'Here, Linz, we'd best have sex again in case I lose!'

Brandon and I were also working together on Paul's image. He was trying to grow his hair by now and one journalist had coined the nickname, 'the Beckham of the Baize'. He was certainly being groomed as one of snooker's big stars but he also had an image as a really nice, straightforward guy who genuinely cared for his fans. He would sign autographs for anybody, anywhere. He always recognized that it was the fans who kept the players where they were, and he had such a lovely nature that he didn't have to fake the friendliness. Whether he won or lost he would always have time for any fans who hung around the snooker hall exits to get a glimpse of their heroes.

One night in Scotland during the BetFred Premier League, he met a fan before the start of a big tournament. The rain was torrential and there was still snow on the ground from earlier that day. Just as Paul arrived at the hotel, after hours of travelling and delays, he noticed a guy who had been waiting to see him for a while. He collared Paul outside the hotel while the weather was still doing its best to keep everyone indoors. Paul chatted to this guy for ages – he was never one to just sign an autograph quickly and then move on. He found out the man's name, what he did for a living, and generally made this guy feel that he had met the real Paul Hunter – who wasn't any different from the public image. The next day as Paul stood at the top of the steps waiting to enter the arena, his name was called out to approach the table. As all of the fans started clapping, Paul took a few steps down and then recognized the guy from outside the hotel the night before. The cameras were rolling and fans were clapping, but Paul shouted out the name of the fan and asked him how he was and if he had managed to get there all right in the terrible weather.

This was typical Paul. He never thought of himself as the great snooker star who was better than anyone else. He had as much time for one individual fan as he did for the corporate millionaires who sometimes paid great wads of cash to play him in private. He was happy to keep everyone waiting, cameras rolling, so that he could make one guy very happy. That was the type of behaviour that made Paul so loved by so many – but of course no one could ever love him more than I did.

Chapter Twelve

Engaged

2001

During the 2000/2001 season, with Brandon onside, Paul Hunter was a force to be reckoned with at the age of just 22. He reached the quarter-finals, semi-finals and finals of so many tournaments. He was a runner-up at the Regal Welsh Open, a semi-finalist at the British Open and a semi-finalist at the Regal Scottish Open. Alan continued to go with Paul to all the competitions, as he had done before Brandon came on the scene. Alan loved the game and got on with everyone on the circuit. It therefore became his responsibility to entertain sponsors and friends at the bar, and Paul gave him the honorary title of 'Head of the Entertainments Committee'. As long as he was near his son, watching him playing snooker, Alan was happy.

Meanwhile, Paul's and my relationship just got better and better as well. It's funny to find out later what other people were thinking about you at the time. Now that Paul's gone, his parents have both said that they were convinced I was right for him from the start. Alan says he noticed that I had a great calming effect on Paul, and that he and Kris knew their son needed someone grounded like me to look after him. And once Paul himself resolved to start getting his life in order, I think he knew that this was the real thing.

In March 2001, Paul was getting ready to fly out to the Chinese Open, so we decided to go for a nice meal together a couple of days before he left. I tended to drive us around so that Paul could have a drink, so that night I went to collect him from his mum and dad's house. Leanne was there, and Nicky was giving his mum an aromatherapy massage.

As soon as I came into the house, Paul shouted that he was upstairs. I went up to his room, and he pushed the door closed behind me. 'Paul!' I said, 'What are you doing?' He was playing 'Whole Again' by Atomic Kitten, and he picked me up and spun me round in the air. I just thought he was being daft but then he put his hand into the top pocket of his denim jacket and pulled out a box. 'What do you think of that, then?' he asked me.

I was baffled. 'What? What do I think of what?' He opened the box and, still baffled, I asked him, 'What is it?' He had this big grin all over his face, as though he had done something really clever. 'It's an engagement ring! I want us to get engaged!' I shrieked and grabbed hold of him and picked *him* up. I was so giddy with happiness, I didn't know what I was doing. He said later that he didn't know where I'd got my strength from.

I wanted to know if he'd asked my dad's permission – I like everything done properly – but he hadn't. I could let that pass. 'Do you want to get engaged?' he asked me, quite worried. I realized that I hadn't given him an answer yet. 'Of course I do! Of course I do!' I told him.

We were both shaking so much that we could hardly fit the ring on my finger. It was just perfect – a perfect fit and a perfect shape. Paul had designed it himself, with a little bit of help from Nicky. There was a single diamond with a solid bit on either side of the stone. 'I went into the jewellers and told them what I wanted,' said Paul. 'When I went back to get it a few days later, I thought they'd made a mistake – it's so tiny I never thought it would fit you.' It was like a dream come true. 'It's gorgeous,' I told him, 'but I'd have been happy with one from a Kinder egg.' I planned never to take it off – it was a symbol of how close we were and how much closer we would become over the years. Of course, I thought then that we had our whole lives ahead of us. I imagined looking at that same ring when we were both grey-haired and playing with our grandchildren. I couldn't envisage anything ever taking that ring, and what it meant, away from me.

Paul had discussed it with his mum, Leanne and Nicky. They came in to congratulate us and told me that he had been so excited earlier on he couldn't decide what to do. 'Should I give the ring to Lindsey straight away and ask her to get engaged,' he'd asked them, 'or wait until we've had the meal and present it to her then?' They had all agreed – wait until after the meal and then surprise me. They should have known that while Paul had patience if he needed it at the snooker table, he didn't have it in any other part of his life. That's why he'd pretty much proposed as soon as I walked in the door. He couldn't hold out. 'I was definitely going to wait until the end of the meal,' he admitted, 'but I could feel that bloody box in my pocket and thought I was going to be sick with nerves. I couldn't wait until the end of the meal, because I couldn't have eaten anything anyway!' It turned out that I was the one who felt sick with excitement when we finally did go out, and I could hardly eat a thing.

We went to one of our favourite restaurants in Leeds and, although we didn't talk about the engagement constantly, I twirled my diamond all night. I knew that we weren't going to get married immediately as Paul needed to calm down. 'I think long engagements are a good idea,' he said as we ate. 'And I don't really want to get married until I'm about 30 anyway.' Thirty? He was only 21. I'd need to get a few things straight right away. 'No, Paul,' I told him. 'That's not the plan at all. If we're engaged, we're engaged to get married; married long before you turn 30.'

He did manage to hold out a bit longer, though – three years and two months to be precise.

I wasn't worried. I knew that getting engaged was a huge step for him and I didn't want to push him any further. I always had to strike the right balance with Paul. The one thing we did chat about that night was the idea of him moving into my house with me. My mum and dad had never liked the idea of their girls living with someone until they were engaged, but I knew they wouldn't mind now that I had a ring on my finger.

I asked Paul again if he would speak to my dad to ask his permission but he didn't see why he should. He said that it was an old-fashioned thing to do and that my dad would be fine about it. I wasn't so sure – Dad liked things done the 'proper' way, and although my parents adored Paul, he would earn even more future son-in-law gold stars if he went about this the way they would appreciate.

We went back to Kris and Alan's to stay the night. At about 3am, I woke up with a start. I saw Paul lying beside me and remembered what had happened. Had I been dreaming? Slowly, I moved one hand towards the other. I closed my eyes and checked my engagement finger just to make sure – it was there, it was still there! My gorgeous twinkling diamond ring was in place, looking as if it was the most natural thing in the world. It was all true – that was my fiancé lying next to me.

Only one thing niggled and as soon as I got up in the morning, I rang Dad to say that Paul had asked me to get engaged. 'Is that all right?' I asked him. He paused, then said, 'If that's what you want, it's fine by me,' and that was that. I would have liked it all to be 'by the book' – and I know Dad would have too – but Paul never understood how I felt about doing things the right way, and the only thing that really mattered was that it worked out fine in the end.

I went back into work that Monday and I was glowing. I showed everyone my ring and told them how happy I was, but I bet a few of them were wondering if it would last or if we'd even get to the wedding stage, given how on and off Paul and I had been for such a long time. But we were deliriously happy.

Paul went to the Chinese Open and reached the quarter-finals, and when he got back we spent all the time we could together, between tournaments. I was blown away by him – each moment I spent with him was happy. He was still as cheeky as ever, teasing me about all sorts of things: he teased me about being 'middle class'; about being too sensible and forward-thinking; and about the fact that I was allowed to wear sexy clothes, but only for him. Paul made me laugh at myself, which was good for me. Sometimes people would be shocked if they heard him saying things like 'Go make us a bacon sandwich, you old tart!', but it was a running joke between us because it was the complete opposite to my straight-laced manner. He would always say things with a twinkle in his eye if he knew he was pushing his luck and I always saw the funny side. It was his cheekiness that got me hooked on him in the first place and it always made me smile.

About four months after we were engaged, I made a suggestion. 'Paul,' I said, 'it's about time you got yourself some responsibility.' He smiled at me. 'Shall I get a goldfish, Lindsey?' he asked.

'No,' I answered, 'but you should get yourself a flat or a house. You've got the money, you need to start learning to pay bills and looking after yourself.'

Paul lived in a world where everyone adored him and he never had to lift a finger apart from at the snooker table. I don't think Paul ever felt grown up – and why would he? It's not a realistic experience being a professional sportsman. So much is done for them, and they're part of a celebrity world that encourages them to think they're not like other people. Paul wasn't yet getting as much media coverage as he would in the future, but he was known; and, even though he was a lovely lad who didn't have any airs and graces, if he had worked in a regular job, he would have had a more responsible attitude. I just wanted him to realize that he couldn't take things for granted. He needed to learn that you could get a lot of pleasure out of knowing that you'd done something for yourself. I had been thinking for a while that someone of Paul's age, with his earning potential, should have his own house. With Brandon's help, he took on the lease of a lovely little cottage in summer 2001 and his sister Leanne moved in with him. He didn't spend much time there, though, because most nights he was staying with me by this time.

A couple of months after that, Paul went out for the night but told me he wouldn't be late. Midnight came and went and he hadn't turned up. Other people might worry that he'd had an accident or think he might be lying drunk in a gutter somewhere, but there was only one explanation that sprang into my mind – Gemma.

As far as I was aware, they hadn't seen each other for ages. Of course, because we all lived in Leeds, we would sometimes bump into her on a night out, but nothing more than a strained 'hello' would be said. I knew she had a new boyfriend by then, but I had no idea if it was serious or not.

I kept calling Paul's mobile, but it was switched off.

I called Anthony, but his was switched off too.

I called Nicky, but she was out with her boyfriend Nobby and didn't know what her little cousin was up to.

I didn't really need any of them to tell me what my gut

knew. He was with her. I just felt it. I sat in an armchair in my pyjamas until about four in the morning. I remembered all the other times I'd sat there, wondering where he was, knowing where he was. This time, I wasn't going to try and find his car, I wasn't going to spy on Paul, I'd just wait – which I did until he fell in the door just as morning was breaking, obviously the worse for wear.

He saw me sitting there as soon as he came in and staggered over. He took my hand and started to say something, some excuse, some explanation. 'Paul,' I said, looking him straight in the eye, 'You don't have to explain. You were with Gemma, weren't you?' He nodded and started to witter on about bumping into her, and about her saying she'd missed him. 'It doesn't matter,' I said.

'Really, Linz? Really?' As he said it, there was relief in his eyes. I could have felt sorry for him but I knew I had to stand firm.

'I don't care,' I lied. 'Just do me two little favours.'

'Anything, Linz.'

'Give me my sodding keys back and take this …' I threw my engagement ring at him, 'when you leave!'

He looked shocked and scrambled around on the floor to find the ring.

'Go. Now. You'll never do this to me again, Paul Hunter. Never.'

I stormed into my bedroom and locked the door, feeling utterly devastated. Even through his drunkenness, Paul must have realized how serious I was because he did collect his things and leave.

Nicky called me the next morning, a few hours after Paul had left. 'Lindsey? What's happened between you and our Paul?'

'How much do you know?' I asked her.

'Enough to realize he must have been stupid again. He came to ours in the early hours of the morning in such a state. He slept in the spare room and I only got bits of the story when he surfaced for something to eat.'

'It's pretty straightforward, Nicky. One word. Gemma.'

'No!' she exclaimed. 'Not again? I thought that was all done and dusted?'

'So did I,' I admitted, 'but it obviously isn't. She must have something I don't because he just doesn't seem to be able to keep away from her. I think that—'

I didn't get to finish my sentence because Paul grabbed the phone from Nicky's hand. 'Lindsey, babes,' he started to say, 'I can explain.'

'No, you can't, Paul. I don't want you to even try, because how could I believe a word of it?' I slammed the phone down and unplugged it from the wall socket, and turned my mobile off too. I was completely determined that day – as determined as any of the hundred other times I'd sworn Paul would never get back into my life after cheating. But he was determined too. There were flowers. There were messages. There were letters. Brandon phoned me. Nicky phoned me. Leanne phoned me. Paul's mum phoned me. All of them said the same thing – that I was the one for him and he would be mad to let me go.

I gave in.

Of course I gave in. I was in pieces and missing him really badly. Still, I held out for two weeks before I agreed to meet him for a drink after work to talk about things. I had to hold myself back when I saw him; he looked so gorgeous even though he was just in jeans and a t-shirt. His blond hair had been growing for a while, and it made him look more handsome than ever. I pulled myself together and walked over to where he was waiting.

'Lindsey, thanks for meeting me. I appreciate it,' he began formally. He couldn't stay serious for long, though. 'Shall we just go back to yours? It's always better making up than falling out.'

God, he had a nerve! Still, he'd broken the ice and I felt relaxed with him as we went to the pub.

'I don't really know what to say.' Paul began as soon as we sat down. 'It was mad of me – I'm a danger to myself sometimes. I know that it's you I want to be with and I know that I've mucked it up. Please can I have one last chance?'

'You've had a lot of those, Paul.'

'OK – can I have one first chance? What happened with Gemma – that was it. My final fling. You've ruined me for anyone else. I want us to be together, I want that to be the last time I hurt you – I want it to all start from now. You and me. Forever.'

'There's something I want to say too, Paul,' I told him. 'You can go and look for someone else as much as you want. You can search high and low. And if you find someone, good luck to you. But I know you will never, ever find someone who loves you and takes care of you the way I do. If there is such a girl out there, you grab her because she'll be bloody amazing.'

'I mean it, Linz. I don't want anyone else ever again for the rest of my life. Only you.' He looked so sad that I decided to put him out of his misery and let him know he was forgiven.

We were set from then on. It was as if what had happened was his final fling, just as he had said. He stopped running after other women and grew up. We were solid. So was Gemma – I heard on the grapevine that she found someone else, settled down and had a baby not long afterwards. Finally, we were all getting on with our lives.

Paul and I played very different roles in our relationship. I never minded looking after him. He wasn't exactly a 'new man', as I found out while we were living together. If he ever attempted any DIY, you could guarantee it would end in disaster, with things in a worse state than when he began. He wasn't technology-friendly either. When we got a laptop it took him ages to even ask how to work it – eventually, he was really chuffed when he knew how to turn it on. I was the one who dealt with anything practical around the house, and took care of the housework and cooking as well.

Our lifestyle was a mixture of the mundane stuff that all couples do and some completely mad stuff. I remember we got invited to London to the premiere of the film *Seabiscuit.* A lot of my memories are based on hairstyles; Paul's was long at that time and it was before I got my hair extensions. I wanted to find something posh to wear as it was going to be a red carpet do, but in the event, I managed to get a lovely black dress from Top Shop for £20. I couldn't believe it when I saw us pictured in *Hello!* and I was wearing a cheap frock. They didn't know what else was going on, that's for sure. I had bought some tights from Debenhams, not fishnets exactly but full of holes like cobwebs. They were really stretchy and when we were in the hotel, it was a nightmare to get them on. So, I was wearing my Top Shop dress and a little shoulder shrug and my bargain shoes and the stretchiest tights in the world. We walked up the carpet – there were so many people there, so many photographers shouting 'Paul!' and 'Lindsey!' They must have done their homework because I'm sure they'd never seen me in their lives before. Surely they should have been concentrating on the stars of the movie like Tobey Maguire?

I heard someone shout, 'Paul, go get Lindsey!' and I realized that I was lagging behind him. I couldn't walk quickly because those bloody tights were all droopy and hanging down my crotch by this time. They were shrinking back to their normal size and I was on a red carpet surrounded by famous people. I was a bit in awe to even be there but my tights brought me back down to earth.

People always thought we'd be at loads of events, but we weren't really. I preferred snuggling up on the sofa with Paul watching his soaps; it was always a bad day for him if he missed *Coronation Street*. It must be different if you do nothing, but I had a job so I couldn't just follow Paul round everywhere at the drop of a hat. I had my own life. I'm not saying anything against all these wives and girlfriends of footballers and other sportsmen, but it would drive me mad to do nothing but shop all day. I like working. I'd work no matter what, and Paul respected that.

We were also lucky in that we had so many friends, friends we'd had for ages. We didn't need any more, so there was never the opportunity for fairweather friends to sneak in as Paul got more and more famous. We stuck with the old crowd who'd been around before.

In summer 2001, we had our first holiday as a couple at a place called the Banyan Tree in Phuket, Thailand. It was one of the nicest holidays ever, Paul and I agreed. We spent two whole weeks together and were never more than two metres apart from each other the whole time. We had a private villa with our own pool and outdoor jacuzzi, where we could stay hidden behind the walls, getting massaged by Thai women with incredibly strong thumbs. Some evenings we went out into the town of Patong, where I was shocked to see the lady boys with no knickers dancing on tables. I'd never come across that kind of thing before but Paul had been to Bangkok and wasn't quite so surprised. We also had fun exploring the shops and markets looking for furniture for our new house. Paul and I loved travelling and this was just the first of a number of lovely holidays we had together. Whenever we had the chance during breaks in the snooker season we took off abroad – a romantic trip to Paris or a hot, exotic holiday to Jamaica. Paul loved anywhere with a beach or pool. They were wonderful times.

When I told clients I was engaged, they'd ask what my boyfriend did for a living. I'd say, 'He's in snooker,' and they'd ask, 'What do you mean?' It was exactly the question I would once have asked. What does 'in snooker' mean? They might have assumed I meant he made tables, or sold cues, or was a cameraman on telly. They'd say, 'Is he famous?' and I'd reply, 'If you watch snooker you'll probably know him, but if you don't, you won't.' I wasn't bothered. If they said they watched snooker, I'd tell them his name was Paul and they'd usually screech, 'Is it Paul Hunter? You're getting married to *him?*'

If you only see someone on telly you probably think they live in a different world, but it's only different if you want it to be. People were surprised when they saw Paul and me doing normal, everyday stuff. Why? Should we have had servants? It wasn't often that I could get him to come to the supermarket with me, but when I did people would ask him for his autograph while we were buying bread and spuds. We only had a tiny bit of that kind of attention but it must become awful when you get it constantly wherever you are, to have your own life taken away because everyone recognizes you. Paul and I would never let it get out of hand – you don't have to take every bit of media attention you're offered.

Paul was doing his job and I was doing mine – and part of mine was to look after him. Thankfully, I had Brandon helping alongside me, and things were just getting better and better for us.

After beating Fergal O'Brien in the 2001 Wembley Masters, Paul secured his place as one of snooker's greats in 2002. He won his second Regal Welsh Open title in January 2002, getting revenge over Ken Doherty, who had beaten him 9–2 in the previous year's final. He then went on to win his second Masters in February – only the third player ever to defend the title successfully; and then at the 2002 British Open, he captured his second ranking title that year. By that stage, having won three major trophies in one year, Paul was up to a world ranking of 9.

We had decided it was time to buy a place together as two separate places didn't really work. Paul was hardly ever at his cottage – we spent most of our time at mine. But every time we went to view a new house, Paul would find something wrong with it even if it was lovely – he was really fussy about houses. One day, we picked up a new batch of property details and a particular house just jumped out at us. Detached with electric gates and five bedrooms, it was on the outskirts of Leeds in a leafy suburb called Batley. As soon as Paul went for a viewing he wanted to buy it.

'This is it, Linz,' he said, squeezing my hand. 'This is where we'll spend the rest of our lives.' The day he paid £350,000 mortgage-free for that house was one of the happiest days of his life. We took a taxi to Batley and, as we didn't have the keys yet, stood holding onto the electric gates for 10 minutes. Paul was so happy he was crying, God bless him.

We moved in to Batley in April 2002 and it was soon a fantastic home. We created a games room where Paul had his own pool table, dartboard, fruit machine, jukebox and a bar with optics where he could serve drinks for his friends. There was plenty of space for people to stay over if they wanted, and I liked to keep 'open house' for anyone to drop in when they felt like it. We had some great parties there and some very happy times. Of course, we had no idea then about the madness that lay waiting for us just around the corner.

Chapter Thirteen

Wedding plans

2002–2003

All the journalists and photographers who followed Paul's career must have thought they'd still be doing stories about him until he retired. His illness must have affected them too; it must have brought home to lots of other professionals just how fleeting everything can be. The only permanence we have is what we leave behind – and Paul didn't just leave a sporting legacy, he left a living one: this bouncy little girl with his looks who is chattering away as I sit here packing up our belongings in order to move, and fighting back the tears. The way Paul looks in that famous Plan B photo is the way he looked when we moved on to the next stage of our lives.

In summer 2002, Paul went to a charity auction. Brandon was trying to raise his profile by making sure he was seen at lots of events at different places. Needless to say, Paul got roaring drunk and put in tons of silly bids for things. Thankfully, we didn't end up with the back end of a racehorse or a timeshare in some place we'd never heard of. He actually did well and got us a holiday in Jamaica. I never found out how much he paid for it – probably a small fortune – but we were both very excited about it as the week of the holiday approached in October that year.

Paul was so pleased with himself, he kept telling me all the details even though he'd read the information from the same travel pack that I'd been reading too. 'It's in a golf resort, Lindsey,' he'd say. 'But we don't have to play golf all the time. There's all sorts of stuff for you too – facials … and nails … and stuff.' I always had to laugh when Paul tried to work out what would interest me. He got the same panicked look in his eyes as he did around Christmas and my birthday. Bless him – all he could think I might want to do was exactly the same stuff I spent my working life doing. Still, it would be nice to be on the receiving end for a change, and I looked forward to spending some time alone with him.

We had a wonderful time in Montego Bay. The people were friendly and welcoming from the moment we stepped off the plane, and the lifestyle of sitting on the beach and having a drink in the sun was one that Paul and I felt we could easily get used to. It was just complete relaxation from the first day to the last. All around us were other couples who didn't look quite so relaxed when they first arrived and we soon worked out why. These were the bridal parties who had decided to get wed in Jamaica. There were people being driven to their wedding ceremonies in golf buggies covered in flowers. The brides looked so beautiful in all their different dresses adapted for beach weddings and, after the services, everyone seemed relaxed and happy. Paul noticed all of this too.

'Here, Lindsey,' he said one day from his sun lounger, 'I think we should do it.'

'What's that, babes?' I asked lazily.

'Get married.'

'We will – we're engaged. Anyway, didn't you say you wanted to wait until you are 30?' I teased him.

'I've changed my mind,' he said excitedly, sitting up. 'I want to get married soon. Abroad. Here. I want us to get married here, Linz!'

I told him that it was the bride's prerogative to decide where and when, but he started tickling me, just as he used to do way back when he was a teenager and we were all in Nicky's bedroom. I could never resist when he did that, and soon I was agreeing, anything to stop the tears of laughter running down my face.

Actually, his plan did make sense. Paul had a huge family and that was partly behind his reasoning; he didn't want hundreds of people there, just a select few. I didn't have a lot of family, nowhere near as many as him, so it seemed like a great idea to me. We left it at that, just as an idea in the back of our minds, but as the holiday went on, we watched a few more of these weddings and everybody seemed so happy, so relaxed, that it was starting to seem like a perfect plan to me too. Paul would say, 'Look, Lindsey, there goes another one. Look at the smiles on them. Look how happy they are.' He was exaggerating it all, but there was no need – I was coming round to the idea anyway.

One night we went to a trendy reggae bar called Rick's Café that was reached by following a bumpy track through some woods, and we started talking it over again. It turned out that we'd both been deciding separately that, behind all the joking, we were keen on a Jamaican wedding. Paul called Brandon that night and told him what we wanted, asking him what he thought. It wasn't exactly a career issue, but Brandon had become a wise friend and confidant and we wanted his opinion. Fortunately, Brandon was all for it as well and it was great to have him on side.

I wanted us to do this, and for our wedding to be a bit different, but I could see there would be a bit of a problem because there were so many people we wanted to invite and who would want to come. If we were getting married thousands of miles from Leeds it simply wouldn't be an option for lots of them. I called my parents and told them what we were planning and they thought it was a great idea, but when Paul phoned home to his mum and dad, Kris was initially very upset. She said there were lots of relatives on their side who would want to be there but who couldn't travel or couldn't afford it.

I couldn't blame her for bringing it up as we'd considered all those same questions ourselves. How would we manage it? Would people be willing or even able to go abroad? Would we pay for them all? What about the people who couldn't make it?

Paul and I kept going back to the reggae bar that we had found, which had become our place for discussions. New ideas kept going through my head and one night I suggested to him how we could solve everything: we'd have two weddings. We'd do the main one for close family and close friends in

Jamaica, where the setting was absolutely idyllic, and then we'd have a reception back home in Leeds afterwards. That way nobody would feel left out and nobody would feel obliged to come to Jamaica if they couldn't afford it or didn't fancy it.

I was sure it would all work out, but when we phoned Brandon again, he began to voice a few concerns. He'd been thinking about it and was worried about the 'logistics'. Brandon and his logistics! He brought up issues such as the weather – how would we control that? What if it was too hot? What if it rained? How would we actually have a wedding on the beach anyway? He said that he had been on holidays where a large number of people mixed and it was always difficult to make sure everyone got on. He said that when it was a wedding and a family background was thrown into the mix, it would be even harder.

'Brandon,' I said, 'it's our wedding and it will be perfect. This is what we want. We're not doing it for other people; we're doing it for us. If anyone has a problem, they shouldn't come. If it rains, we'll get umbrellas. If it's too hot, we'll put more sun cream on.'

Paul and I wouldn't have our minds changed by anyone. We were carried away by the seven-mile beach and glorious weather, but Brandon was right about one thing – it would be a lot to organize. By the time we left Jamaica, Paul and I were convinced we would be coming back to become husband and wife – and we were both prepared to argue with anyone back in Leeds who tried to convince us otherwise. We were a team on this, and heaven help anyone who tried to steer us off course.

We were met at the airport on our return home by Brandon and Charlotte. Maybe Charlotte had been working on Brandon, because by now he was as excited as we were. It was going to be a lot to organize but Brandon knew a woman called Diane who was a wedding organizer, and she was going to turn out to be a godsend. About six weeks after Paul and I got back from Jamaica, I met up with her to talk about what we liked and what the options were. There were three hotels in the complex we had chosen, one of which had facilities for children, which we were keen on since there were lots of children in the family. Diane suggested that we have a bit of a do on the beach and then go to Rick's Café afterwards, the place Paul and I had visited when we first made our decision to have the wedding in Jamaica. Diane also suggested we hired a catamaran to get there. It was right on the edge of a cliff and there weren't any main roads to it. When Paul and I had been there, we'd had a bumpy journey through woods and it took over an hour even though it was only 15 minutes away as the crow flies. We didn't want all the guests to have to do that so the catamaran sounded like a good idea.

Diane did a terrific job helping us to plan it all so well before we even got there. It was quite a big undertaking because there turned out to be 26 guests in the end – not necessarily all the people who were absolutely closest to us, because it depended on who could afford it. Sadly, my cousin Helen couldn't make it, the one I had stood up for when she was bullied at school; she had been travelling the world for a year and was far too skint to get to Jamaica.

The plans went on for months. I was exhausted by the end of it as there were so many things to arrange, but once the decision had been made, Paul and I never wavered from the notion of getting married in Jamaica. Kris wasn't the only one to voice her concerns, but I told them all that the wedding was for us, not anybody else, and we wanted it this way.

The idea of having a second wedding calmed them all down too. Paul had a sponsor called Bredbury Hall, a hotel run by Brandon's best friend. The owner said he would let us have the whole hotel to ourselves on the Sunday night when we came back from Jamaica, as the Monday was a bank holiday. That seemed like a good idea. The following week, he got back to us again and said we could have a meal during the day as well, so we ended up planning two proper wedding days. Jamaica would be an amazing, relaxed day, then we'd come back to Manchester for a do for everybody else. We hadn't planned to spend a fortune on the second wedding, but it soon became clear that it would snowball into a huge fantastic day.

I'd never been happier. I had to keep pinching myself. I was getting married to the man I adored – how lucky was I? Those days were magical, and I can still see it all as if it was yesterday. It doesn't make me sad; how could it? We were living a dream life.

In the year running up to the wedding, Paul was becoming more well known in the wider world of sport. By then 1970s and 1980s smash BBC TV programme *Superstars* had been recommissioned, in which sportsmen from all different professions get together to see who is the best at a variety of different sports. Paul was invited to appear on the show, which was being filmed in La Manga, Spain, in May 2003. Although reticent at first, he decided to give it a go – not because it would raise his profile, but because it might be 'a laugh'. Typical Paul. When we got there, the meeting room was full of sports stars, including Ricky Hatton, the boxer; Stuart Pearce, the England football captain; and rugby player Gavin Hastings. Some of the competitors of Paul's age were very fit and there to win. These people were proper athletes, whereas Paul didn't even walk to the end of the drive if his car was handy, so he was a bit apprehensive about appearing in skintight black lycra alongside them all.

The organizers explained that there would be running, swimming, field sports, all sorts of competitions, before the winner would be announced. 'Bloody hell,' said Paul, 'I thought it would just be a piss up!' Hardly – the others thought that a glass of wine a week was pushing the boat out. Paul would go down for training when he felt like it, usually with a fag in one hand and a drink in the other. Rather than think this was terrible behaviour, the others took a shine to him and he was nominated to be the entertainments director, a job he loved. He did manage to get a few of them to drink – but not much, so he was generally left with full jugs of sangria each night.

His performance in the show wasn't as bad as it could have been. He came third in the 100 metres, beating Gavin Hastings, and third at football, and he held his own in golf –

but everyone was proud of him because he always tried his hardest, even when he was falling down at the end of it. I think most of the other guys looked on him as a little brother figure, and they were all really friendly. The show was televised later that year in October and gave us a good laugh.

In the 2003/2004 season Paul reached number 8 in the world rankings. The match that really got him recognized was the 2004 Masters when two of the biggest personalities in the game were set for a match that would go down in snooker history.

Paul wasn't the only character in the game at this time. Ronnie 'the Rocket' O'Sullivan had his own army of fans, and although Ronnie's character was different from Paul's (he often suffered from depression), he was also an absolute genius at the table. Paul got on well with him – Paul got on with everyone; there was no doubt that their attitudes were chalk and cheese and yet there was ultimate respect for each other's achievements.

When they appeared at the top of the steps to walk down to that table at Wembley in February 2004, the crowd went wild. It wasn't like snooker – it was as if two pop stars were going head-to-head in a boxing match.

Paul trailed Ronnie throughout most of the match – 2–0, then 6–1, then 7–2, then 8–6, before staring defeat in the eye at 9–7 to Ronnie. The title would go to the first player to reach 10. Television schedules were rearranged and it seemed as if the whole of the UK was staying up to watch this epic battle. I was there and I was terrified. I had told Paul so often that it didn't matter if he won or lost, but I knew he wanted this one badly, even if it didn't show in his demeanour.

Maybe the millions of viewers were willing him on, maybe some part of him had an inkling that it would be his last grandstand appearance before his world turned upside down, or maybe he was just brilliant. Whatever the reason, Paul won the last three frames to claim the sixth major title of his professional career. He was at that time only the third player to have won three Masters titles – but Ronnie has since equalled his record.

That victory had him walking on air for the whole of the year and he finished the season with his highest-ever world ranking of 4.

Even when he lost, he didn't mind as it was often his friends who were the winners and Paul could be as happy for them as he was for himself. In the 2004 Daily Record Players Championship in April, he had almost achieved one of his famous comebacks but his great friend Jimmy White narrowly won the title. As it was Jimmy's first ranking title in almost 12 years, Paul was as happy for him as he would have been for himself. Jimmy's dad ran out and the three of them – Paul, Jimmy and his dad – were hugging and kissing, jumping up and down. You'd hardly think Paul had just lost £70,000 and the LG Order of Merit! He couldn't have been more delighted for his mate!

Personal happiness and professional success were all coming together for Paul, and he was glorying in it. He couldn't put a foot wrong – everywhere people were clamouring for more and more of Paul Hunter. He didn't need success to be happy, but he loved the way he could make others happy and proud of him.

And he certainly did.

Paul and I were getting very close to Brandon and Charlotte, and by now they were more like friends than business acquaintances. We had decided it would be a nice gesture to get married on their wedding anniversary on 19th May 2004. At one point, Brandon and Charlotte even thought about renewing their vows on the same day, but Brandon got worried about the 'logistics' as usual. Who would look after their kids while they got 'wed'? Who would take over dealing with any problems if Brandon was busy with his own ceremony? Eventually we decided it would just be Paul's and my day, but it was even more special knowing that the date meant something to Brandon and Charlotte as well.

One night the four of us were out for a meal together in Leeds when Paul got distracted by some fans who wanted autographs and photos. He went over to their table and the three of us were left alone.

'Do you know, Lindsey,' said Brandon, 'I wasn't sure I'd ever see this day. When I first met you, I was expecting the usual snooker girlfriend – young, daft and out for a good time on the back of her boyfriend's talent.'

'You should have told me, Brandon. I'd have been happy to knock those ideas out of your head,' I joked.

'You did, you did – pretty much straight away,' he said. 'Paul thought he would never be tamed, but I always knew, from the minute I met you, that if any woman could do it, it would be you. I think that you've got a lot to be proud of, Lindsey Fell.'

'I love Paul. I've always loved Paul, and I've always known we were right for each other. It wasn't about me taming him, Brandon, it's always just been about us being together as I knew we should be from the start.'

'Talking about me again?' said Paul when he came back to the table.

'As always, babes, as always.' I laughed – but the truth was, we usually were. We all loved Paul so much and we all wanted the best for him; I hoped he knew that.

Paul and I were in the media quite a lot by this time, so people assumed we would get a magazine deal to cover the wedding. In fact, I was never very keen on this because I didn't want to lose control of the day. You always run the risk of magazines bossing you around, deciding what you should do, what photos should be taken, even whether guests are allowed to have their own cameras or not, and that worried me. However, Brandon said it would be good for Paul's profile if it came off so we went along with it for a while.

Brandon got into initial discussions with some of the celebrity magazines but he always had the figure of £30,000 in his head and wasn't going to do a deal for less. Apparently some of them were really snooty, talking down their noses to him and telling him that 'snooker doesn't sell magazines'. It was as if they had a notion that all snooker fans watch

Coronation Street and keep whippets and are too lowbrow to read magazines. Brandon said their ignorance made him laugh but I think he was secretly very annoyed. By the start of 2004, Paul was famous internationally. He was making a huge impact by taking part in promotional matches in China, Germany, Ireland and all over Europe. He travelled everywhere to further the game whenever the snooker authorities and his manager asked him to go. After winning the epic Masters in February 2004, Paul was even more recognizable but he was a genuine person who wasn't interested in commerciality or fame as such.

In the end, I decided to hire a photographer who worked freelance for *Hello!* magazine to take our wedding photos but in a private contract between him and us. I was very relieved that no magazine got to have a say in how my wedding day was run. I didn't need a magazine to tell me how wonderful it all was. I already felt like I was getting ready to marry my Prince Charming – it was a fairy tale come true.

Now I had to turn my mind to a very important matter. All princesses need a special dress, and I was on a mission to find mine.

Chapter Fourteen

Shorter, tighter, better!

2003–2004

I had started looking for a dress about six months before the wedding, but nothing was quite right. I had a picture in my mind of what I wanted but everything I tried on was wrong, just not 'me'. I didn't want a full-length dress; I wanted a split in it or something like that to show off my legs. I didn't want anything too big or too full because I was getting married abroad and I'd have to take it with me on the plane. I traipsed round dozens of shops with Nicky, who was going to be my bridesmaid. Every dress I tried on seemed too flouncy, too fussy. I would hold them up at the front, or shift them around, saying, 'I want it like this, Nicky.'

She'd agree I was right but we just couldn't find anything. 'That style does suit you, Linz,' she'd agree. 'You look better showing your legs off, but you just don't see wedding dresses like that. Wedding dresses are usually a bit conservative but I can't imagine Paul wanting to see you all covered up.' She was right – Paul's idea of a dress was as tiny as possible. Sometimes I'd say to the ladies in the shops, 'Can't you cut bits off them?' but they were never keen; it was as though I was insulting them by asking. I wanted to say, 'It's my wedding day, I know what Paul likes, and he'll want me to look sexy, not like some daft frilly doll.'

One day, I went to a very posh shop and was trying on huge dresses just for fun. 'What am I going to do?' I asked the rather la-di-da woman who was meant to be helping me, when it became obvious that there was nothing for me. 'You need someone to make you one, dear,' she announced. Of course I did! Why hadn't I thought of that before? I asked her whether she knew anyone and she said there was a little shop around the corner, hidden away in a quiet bit of town.

I thought she was joking when I first got there because it looked more like a fancy-dress shop than a wedding bou-tique. Maybe she'd sent me on a wild goose chase because I hadn't bought one of her expensive dresses? I knocked on the door and it was opened by a huge woman who told me that I needed an appointment. She must have felt sorry for me, though, because after I'd begged a bit, she let me in. It was run by her and her sister, who was very big too.

When I walked in, there were bolts of fabric lying every-where, in every colour you could imagine, and there was a mangy dog loping around. It hardly seemed like Bride of the Year stuff. 'What do you want, then?' she asked me without any ceremony.

'A dress? Can you make me a dress? My wedding dress?' I ventured. She looked at me as if I was mad. 'Not a problem. What do you want?' I was still looking round at the place. Could this woman really make my dream dress? Her shop looked like a set for a Harry Potter film. And yet, there was something about her that I trusted. All those big fancy shops had nothing I liked, so why couldn't this woman do better? I started to tell her what I was after, haltingly at first, then with more and more confidence as she kept nodding and jotting it all down as if my requests were the most straight-forward in the world.

I said, 'I've got quite a big bust but I don't really want to wear a bra, so I'll need decent support.' She looked like she knew about those sorts of problems herself, so she nodded. 'I want something strapless with little gems and sequins and crystals all over the front.' She kept nodding. 'Could I have the top bit separate, like a bodice? And I want it all in white satin and organza with silver thread running through the skirt.' More nodding. 'And I know this sounds odd, but can I have it long at the back and short at the front? I want to be able to take the long bit off later on, so I need almost a three-piece.' Not a problem. Nods all round. She went off and got some material to show me. 'How about this?' she asked. 'How about a little mini skirt under-neath a full skirt, sort of pushed to the side?' It was perfect; she had taken my idea, such as it was, and known exactly what I wanted!

She was holding little pieces of fabric against me, but there wasn't another dress to model it on. She noted down my measurements, we agreed a price and that was it, I left. I couldn't believe that I was buying a wedding dress that I hadn't seen, not even in a picture. I didn't have to go back for a fitting until January, four months before my wedding, and

I kept saying to Nicky, 'I hope I like it. I hope it's going to fit me. I hope it's going to look all right.'

It didn't really look like much when I next went back but the basic shape was there and it put my mind at rest a little bit. I bought the shoes and a tiara from the same little shop, and we got Nicky a silver basque and skirt with little pieces of diamanté on top that looked beautiful on her.

I next went back to the funny little shop eight weeks later. It was taking the women a long time to sew every crystal on by hand. This time, I could really see it all coming together – the most important dress I would ever buy.

Every time I went, I asked them to make the skirt shorter and tighter because I was thinking about what Paul would like. He only had one way of judging how I dressed: was there a lot of flesh on display? I applied his rule every time I visited the shop. Shorter! Tighter! Sexier! That would make me the bride he wanted to see on 19 May. Eventually, at the last fitting, I said, 'Just an inch shorter and a little bit tighter and it'll be perfect.' That woman was so patient, so talented, that she did it – she made the most gorgeous dress in the world for my wedding to the most wonderful man in the world. It had to be just right – everything about the day had to be just right – because that would be a sign. A sign of how wonderful our marriage and future life together was going to be.

I was to pick the dress up on the Monday and then we would fly out to Jamaica on the Wednesday. I didn't want to risk putting it in my suitcase and checking it in. I wanted to keep it with me in the cabin, so the dressmaker said, 'I'll box it up for you. Come as late as you can so it doesn't crease, but don't worry too much because it's only little and it'll stretch out.' I asked her to put everything we needed in that box – my dress, Nicky's dress, shoes for both of us, tiara, even my knickers – so that I only had one piece of luggage to worry about.

My mum pulled up outside the shop on the Monday and when I emerged with a little box with a ribbon tied round it to make a handle, she laughed. 'Are you sure it's all in there, our Lindsey? Maybe you've paid £1,600 for an invisible dress!' I said I was sure – but I hadn't actually looked inside so it could have been empty for all I knew.

It was all coming together. The dressmaker said that I should take a single duvet cover with me and cover the dress when we got there. I planned to hang it up in my mum's room because I didn't want anybody to see it before the big day – especially Paul. He wouldn't have been able to resist having a peek if it was in our room.

While I was getting myself into a state about the dress, there were other things to concern me as well. I was having sleepless nights worrying about Paul's stag do. I was scared it would be horrendous and just hoped the lads weren't going to do anything stupid to him that would show in the photos – God forbid that they would shave his head.

I had a great time at my hen do, one weekend in the middle of April. On the Friday night we had a lovely meal in a restaurant in Leeds. My mum and all my friends and some of their parents and my aunties were there. One of Mum's friends gave me a little box as a present. I had to stand up and open it in front of everybody at the restaurant. It contained 'everything the bride needs', with items such as condoms and confetti in an overnight bag. It was so lovely to have lots of women of different ages there, just getting on and enjoying themselves.

The next day, Saturday, three of us had a day of beauty treatments followed by a night out in town. All my friends like different things so I tried to accommodate everyone at some point, and that night was for those who wanted to drink tequila until they couldn't stand. I had a pair of white jeans on and a white top and over these Nicky forced me to wear handcuffs and a sash saying 'wife to be' and all sorts of other bits and pieces. After we were all suitably drunk, we went to a gay bar for more tequila and sambuca slammers and that was when my engagement ring broke for the first time; I must have been slamming too hard. I couldn't believe it. Nicky told me to take it off but I didn't want to. 'I can't do that! Paul will think I've taken it off for a reason,' I wailed. I had to see sense eventually, though, and put it in my handbag.

We went back to one girl's house for nightcaps before I got a taxi back to Nicky's at 5am. When I staggered home in the morning, Paul laughed at the sight of me having trouble walking up the drive. He stood at the front door with his arms crossed, tutting like an old woman. 'Look at the state of you,' he teased. 'You're a disgrace, woman! What time do you call this? You treat this place like a hotel.' He thought he was hilarious but I just had to get to the sofa where I lay for the rest of the day.

The following weekend, the last weekend in April, was Paul's stag do. It was harder for him to schedule a night out because he had to wait until he'd finished in the World Snooker Championships. He had lots of different types of friends too, but they all agreed to start at 2pm at our house with a game of pool and then head into town. Paul could be a party animal at times but there was nowhere he felt more comfortable than at home, so they went into town about 4pm and were back at our house by 10pm. He said he couldn't be bothered painting the town red so they'd all just come back.

Paul was especially happy that Darren Shaw, who he had asked to be his best man, was there. As Darren lived in Warrington, they didn't see much of each other ordinarily although they were very close and would do anything for each other.

Unfortunately, Darren had pancreatitis and shouldn't have been drinking, but I think he allowed himself a few vodkas that night to keep Paul company and he ended up in hospital. The doctors told him he couldn't travel for a while afterwards so he never got to Jamaica after all. Poor Darren. He didn't have any insurance so he lost all his money. He got to be the best man at Bredbury Hall, though, and Nicky's partner Nobby stepped into the breach in Jamaica.

Looking back, it's funny to think how little I really had to worry about. All the details of the day were insignificant – I'd have married Paul in the local registry office with two strangers as witnesses. I'd have done anything for him, anything at all.

Chapter Fifteen

Mr and Mrs Paul Hunter

19 May 2004

My wedding album is one of the last things to be packed. I'm clutching it as Evie plays amongst the chaos. There is one particularly beautiful picture of Paul and me with the sunset behind us and he looks so golden, so healthy and full of life. I touch his face over and over again as Evie waddles over to me.

'Look darling,' I say to her. 'This is your daddy, Evie Rose, this is your daddy.' She gurgles but she's too young to understand. When will she first realize there's something different about her because her daddy isn't around? I try to draw her back to the pictures but she's off, more interested in her new toys than my memories. My mind isn't so easily distracted. Looking at pictures of us in Jamaica brings so many thoughts and scents and reflections flooding back.

Our wedding is the only holiday I've ever been on for which I've bought a whole new wardrobe. I don't often splash out so that was a big deal for me. Paul's preparations had been a lot more straightforward than mine. He had gone to Birmingham to get his suit made and, because I'd picked a white dress, he said he'd have white linen. However, the tailors told him that cream was better because they could line it more smoothly. I wondered whether white and cream would look odd together, but it was fine on the day. Paul's outfit was pretty much last-minute; it was only finished a couple of days before we were due to fly out. When we picked up his shoes and tie, he was so excited. He said it only felt real once he was holding his wedding outfit.

The whole party was flying out together and we travelled en masse to the airport in a coach. I had to admit to a few nerves about how everyone would get on. I hadn't been on holiday with my parents since I was about 15 and they only went on golfing holidays these days so I hoped they would enjoy spending 10 days on a beach. We all got to the airport, checked in, and had a drink and all the while I made sure my box was never out of my sight.

The airline asked us if we wanted to be upgraded on the flight to Jamaica and back, but I preferred us to stick together on the way out; we would come back first class once we were married. Everyone got on fantastically well on the flight. We made a big fuss of my four-year-old nephew Matthew, who was supposed to be my pageboy. He had a little white linen suit and would have looked adorable, but I promised him that he didn't have to be a pageboy if he didn't want to. In the event, he just wanted to play on the sand. We all checked into our hotels, dropping those with kids off at 'Sandy Bay' first as that was the family resort, and we didn't meet up again until the next day.

On the first day, the Thursday, Paul and I had an appointment with the hotel wedding planner. It was blazing hot at midday and I thought that would be a lovely time to get married. The planner suggested we could have the ceremony in a tiny little white archway or in the stone gazebo in their gardens. We wanted the gazebo as soon as we saw it. There was a wedding in progress at the time and it looked gorgeous.

We always had wonderful holidays, but this one was the icing on the cake. Usually, I'd always been working so hard that I used to completely conk out as soon as we stepped off the plane no matter where we were. Paul always marvelled that I could sleep so much – which was rich coming from him. In Jamaica I had more to do, but I did chill for a lot of the time. Paul seemed to be laughing the entire week, having a great experience. I found it hard to take my eyes off him, he was looking so gorgeous. The thought that I was going to be Mrs Paul Hunter in a few days just blew my mind. I was so proud and excited.

Every moment was completely relaxed for everyone on that holiday. It was all-inclusive, so there were no worries about money and the kids could eat what they wanted when they wanted. We didn't have a riotous time; we were in bed by midnight every night after eating a lovely meal together.

I needn't have worried about my mum and dad – they had a ball. It was on this holiday that Paul decided to make up his own pet names for them. They found it hysterical when he started shouting for 'Mil' and 'Fil', his mother-in-law and father-in-law to be. We met up with the wedding guests every day in one of the many hotels and restaurants or down on the beach, and it was such a fantastic setting that everyone had a great time.

There was just one black cloud on the horizon. Literally. It had started to rain every day at lunchtime. It began on the Thursday at about 2pm, then got a bit earlier every day. I worked out that by the day we were due to get married, the rain should kick off at about midday, our chosen time to be walking down the aisle. We knew it was the rainy season, but we never expected it to interfere with our big moment. I had seen couples having to run back to the hotel in the middle of their ceremony, and I knew I would be devastated if that happened to us. I considered changing the time, but I was a bit superstitious about it, thinking that we should just stick to set plans and not mess with arrangements.

The hotel provided a whole package for the bride and groom, so the day before the wedding Paul and I were taken to the beauty spa. We were given full body massages and lots of other lovely treatments. With my professional experience, I knew we were getting the absolute best of everything, but I was a bit surprised when they threw in something that we don't do in Leeds. Paul and I were covered in all these body oils and lotions then the two women doing the treatments said we would be left alone for 30 minutes 'in private'. They giggled a lot and emphasized that we were going to be married the next day, then left. 'Here,' said Paul, 'Do you think they've heard of Plan B out here as well?'

All we did was laugh and enjoy being together – there

was definitely no sex; we'd had enough of being public about that to last us a lifetime.

We spent the night in separate rooms and when I woke the next morning, the sun was streaming in through my open windows. This would be the last morning I would wake up as Lindsey Fell. From today, I would spend every moment beside the man of my dreams, every moment as Mrs Paul Hunter.

I heard a knocking at my door and opened it to find Nicky, champagne bottle in one hand and our dresses in the other. She shrieked at me and came in. 'Can you believe that you're going to get married today?' she asked. 'And to our Paul? Our little Paul?' We hugged each other and jumped around the room like two little kids on Christmas morning – then, unlike two little kids, we started on the champagne. When we looked at the dresses, they seemed even more gorgeous than we'd remembered. Nicky laid out my wedding outfit while I hopped in the shower. We got made up, did our hair, then put the dresses on. I truly did feel like a princess. The dress was perfect. 'Oh, Lindsey,' said Nicky, 'you're going to make him cry when he sees you like that.' I laughed. 'Fat chance,' I told her.

We spent the rest of the time with my mum, helping her to get ready, and before I knew it, the time had come. Just as I was taking one last glimpse in the mirror and marvelling at how lovely everything was turning out, I heard a roar from outside. Thunder. Then the heavens opened.

'Mum! Nicky!' I screamed. 'It's pouring! What are we going to do?'

'Whatever you do, don't cry,' advised Nicky. 'Don't let your mascara run on top of everything else.'

'It won't matter,' I cried in despair. 'Everything's going to get soaked anyway.'

Mum stepped in to try and calm me down. 'The hotel must deal with this all the time,' she said. 'We've seen it ourselves every day; they'll have a plan.'

'Mum,' I interrupted, 'we've seen the plan. It involves everyone running back to the hotel as quickly as they can, drenched.' I was a bag of nerves, my stomach tying itself in knots as I contemplated my big day being wrecked by the weather.

'Let's go downstairs, collect your flowers and see what they've got to say for themselves,' replied Mum. I didn't hold out much hope, but off we went.

The hotel manager was waiting for us in the foyer, holding out my wedding bouquet. He started to compliment us, saying how 'exquisite' we all looked, but Mum was having none of it.

'That's all very well, but what do you expect us to do about this,' she began, pointing vaguely in the direction of the door to the beach behind us.

'What, Madam?' the manager asked.

'This rain!' she said, nearly shouting at him.

'What rain?' he asked calmly, and we all turned round to point out *exactly* what rain. There was nothing. The sun was out, the rain had stopped, and the only sign it had ever happened was some silver droplets glistening on the flowering bushes lining the pathway to the gazebo.

He laughed as our mouths dropped open. 'You're in

Jamaica now, ladies,' he said. 'Things happen and then they're over quickly.'

My dad was waiting for us at the beginning of the path and, as he saw me in my wedding dress for the first time, he couldn't decide whether to laugh or cry. 'You're beautiful,' he told me. 'You look like a princess. I'm so proud, Lindsey, so proud.' I took his arm, squeezed it, and told him not to start blubbing or he'd set me off too. Mum made her way down to where the seats were positioned – they were on two sides of the beach and, at the front, was a little podium where Paul and I would stand to take our vows.

I started walking down the same route (the aisle, I suppose, although it didn't feel like one), with Dad and Nicky. About a third of the way down, before anyone realized we were there, I stopped. I wanted to look at all this and take it in. The seats were full of people we loved, who had made this very special trip. I could see Brandon and Charlotte with their children Annabelle and Max; Tracy and her husband Chris, with their children Matthew and Eloise playing in the sand; my mum and Paul's parents, and more, all waiting for me. I didn't want to cry at all; I felt I could burst with happiness.

'Right, I'm ready,' I told Dad and off we set. The music began to play and everyone turned around, including Paul. He looked so handsome. His hair was long by then and he looked golden and perfect with the sun shining behind him. I could hardly believe we had made it this far. Sometimes I'd thought we would never reach this day but as I walked down towards Paul, I saw the strangest thing.

Nicky had been right.

Paul was crying.

By the time I got to him, he was shaking like a leaf. 'You all right, babes?' I whispered. He nodded to me. 'Yeah. I just can't believe it. Look at you, look at you!' he whispered back.

He managed to get through the vows without crying too much and by the time the ceremony was over, he had pulled himself together – certainly enough to give me more than the regulation 'you may kiss the bride' smooch. 'Right,' he said. 'That's the soppiness gone, let's have a great time.'

A catamaran took us to a local restaurant for a meal. Champagne was served on board and everyone rolled up their trouser legs and pulled up their skirts to dip their feet in the water. Lots of our wedding photographs were taken on that boat. We must have hundreds of shots and none of them would be out of place in the pages of a glossy magazine. Now those photographs are such a precious memory. Our gift from Brandon was a beautiful album with all the best shots stuck in it. There are so many left over I still don't know what to do with them all.

Speedboats took us from the catamaran to the shore. The restaurant was close to a place where locals and tourists dive off the cliffs into the sea. Of course, lots of the blokes had to try the jump once they had a bit of Dutch courage inside them. Brandon reckoned it must have been a 70- or 80-foot drop, but there were local lads doing it from another section of cliff, covered in trees, that was about another 50 feet higher than that. Fortunately no one was injured while we were there. We also had jet skis and paragliding organized for anyone who needed to burn off a bit more adrenaline after lunch.

Some of the photos shot as the sun was setting take your breath away. The whole day from start to finish was breathtaking; it was everything I'd ever dreamed of. It rained for 10 minutes later on, but that just helped to cool the air and settle the dust.

When we finally all returned to the hotel, everyone was just giddy with happiness – it had rubbed off on all the guests, not just Paul and me. They were all hugging and holding each other, making promises to be friends forever. Paul whispered to me, 'And you'll be Mrs Hunter forever too.' I didn't think about it then, but forever's a long time.

As soon as we got back to Leeds, we had the reception at Bredbury Hall for everyone who hadn't been able to make it to Jamaica. We decorated the whole place beautifully, with fairy lights everywhere and huge plants to make it seem a bit like Jamaica. I got to wear my dress again and everyone else was in their wedding outfits. As Paul and I entered the hall, the announcer asked that everyone cheer for 'Mr and Mrs Paul Hunter' and they all went wild. The whole affair was a lot noisier than Jamaica had been.

There was a song that was very special to Paul and me – 'Amazed', by Lonestar – because it just seemed to sum up everything we felt about each other so we danced to it as everyone shouted their congratulations.

When the song ended, there was lots of cheering. We told

everyone to have a great time and the party started, this time with Darren as best man, as he should have been in the first place. We had an oxygen bar and Jamaican music. We had Tina Turner and George Michael impersonators. We had a cocktail bar and the waiters and waitresses were walking round offering tequila to guests.

Everyone had a ball and, at the end of the night, I felt as if I was surrounded in love, wrapped up safely in everyone's good wishes.

All I could say to myself was that the whole thing was like a fairy story; we were blessed.

Chapter Sixteen

D Day

2–3 March 2005

After we were married that May in 2004, our life went
smoothly for the rest of the year. Paul's career was progressing in leaps and bounds – he made it to the top places of
virtually every tournament he participated in. In September
he went on a promotional tour to China and he was treated
like a pop star, with screaming girls and fans queuing for
hours to see him.

It was just after that, in October 2004, that I flew out to
join Paul in Ireland to celebrate his twenty-sixth birthday.
His friend Jimmy White was there – a generation older than
Paul but someone with whom he had a unique bond. Paul felt
so comfortable with Jimmy who was like an older brother to
him. On tournaments they were always having a laugh
together. Jimmy could be a bit of a lad, to say the least. Paul
was fond of telling the story of when Jimmy went out to buy
a pint of milk and came home two days later after a bender.

We spent a thoroughly raucous evening with Jimmy celebrating Paul's birthday. Unbeknown to us, Jimmy had

arranged a special birthday present for Paul that year. We were sitting in a bar when all of a sudden this half-naked girl started dancing in front of us, writhing around and sitting on Paul's lap. Jimmy had bought him a lap dance! I thought it was hilarious, but I said to Paul: 'Those boobs are fake, babes. At least mine are real.' Afterwards Jimmy had arranged for us to get a stretch limo back to the hotel and as soon as we got in, this black screen came up separating us from the driver and Brandon, who was sitting in the front seat. Never one to pass up an opportunity, Paul thought we should take advantage of our privacy – and who was I to disappoint him on his birthday?

We had some great times in those first nine months of being Mr and Mrs Hunter. Our personal life was fantastic and we had agreed to start trying for a baby.

Just before our first wedding anniversary, I decided to keep a diary. I intended to write down all the little things that happened to us during our second year of married life together. I had never been good at keeping a diary any other time, and in some ways I regretted it. I knew people who had kept a diary since they were kids and, although it must have seemed a chore sometimes, it would be great to have something like that to look back on. So, that was what I decided to do – but along with many other good intentions, I failed at that one straight away. After buying the notebook, I scribbled on the front page: *Our journey just before our first anniversary.* And that was that for a while.

* * *

The only cloud on the horizon was that Paul had been complaining about a pain in his side for a little bit. It was intermittent throughout the last few months of 2004. He'd think about going to the doctor and then it got better so we forgot all about it. Paul had never been 100 per cent healthy – he'd had psoriasis and vitiligo since he was a child, and he wasn't exactly a strapping muscle man.

However, when the pain in his side came back and didn't clear up after two weeks, he went to our GP in February 2005. The GP was immediately worried that it might be related to Paul's appendix and he arranged for us to go to a BUPA hospital a few days later for a consultation (we had private medical insurance). We went home to wait, aware that Paul had a tournament coming up in Ireland around the same time. Something kicked me into starting the diary because I wrote: *I've never felt this happy in my life. Paul and I are so in love, so happy, with no worries. We must be the luckiest people around.*

On 2 March 2005, it was time for the BUPA consultation. There was only one question we were concerned about: was Paul's appendix going to burst? He was pretty much in constant pain by this time and had no idea whether he should even be thinking of travelling to Ireland for the exhibition match he had agreed to play there. After the consultation, we were told to come back the next day for a scan that would, hopefully, tell us just how near to bursting his appendix might be, how much time we had before things got too bad, and what the best treatment would be – in particular, whether he needed immediate surgery.

When I think back, it's poignant how little we knew.

I wrote in my journal for 3 March, the scan day: *Hope he does-n't need his appendix out.* To think that was the sum total of our concerns. We couldn't see further than an appendectomy. Looking at what I've written next, I don't know whether to laugh or cry: *Paul had to drink liquid for an hour before the scan and then he had to have an injection. Poor boy!* An injection. Within months his veins would be so riddled with holes that he'd look like a drug addict. Medical staff would be hitting his arms in the hope of finding one, single, solitary vein that could bear to have another needle stabbed into it. And I was feeling the world had ended that day because he had a full bladder and one needle stuck in him.

At 6.25pm we were called back into the consultant's room to be given the results. We were both thinking that we just wanted to get it over with and find out what was going on and get home for the evening.

'Paul's appendix is fine,' the consultant said, and we glanced at each other and smiled.

The relief was overwhelming – but there was a pause between the specialist saying these words and the next sentence. 'But the scan has shown up six cysts in Paul's abdomen and we'd like to do a biopsy to see what's going on.'

Paul had six cysts and the doctors wanted to do a biopsy.

I felt as if I needed to backtrack. Cysts. Biopsy. What happened to his appendix being our only worry? Paul said it would all work out – he was a 'cysty' person; he'd had some removed from his back at one point and from his testicles. He just had a tendency towards them, in the way that some people always got sinus problems when they had a cold, or others always got bronchitis when they had a cough. Paul was 'cysty'.

We had a week or so to wait, hoping that the biopsy would be fine, that the cysts would be benign – that life could go on, back to being ordinary and perfect again. We thought, prayed, that the journey to normality would begin after the biopsy on 16 March.

When the day finally arrived, we hadn't got much sleep the night before. I'd written in my diary: *7.30am. The dreaded day. Paul panicking a little. He keeps saying, 'God, I feel sick.'*

When we got to the hospital, Paul was whisked away and I sat waiting for two hours for him to return from the operating theatre. He finally got back at 11.30am and looked like death warmed up. Of course, I had no idea then how bad he would look in a few months' time. In comparison to that, he was the picture of health. He had been violently sick after the operation and his throat was really sore from the breathing tube that had been stuck down it. I absolutely hate feeling helpless in any situation and I nearly passed out at the thought of how bad Paul felt.

We got home at 4pm and Paul's stomach was very swollen because during the procedure, known medically as a laparoscopy, they had pumped his abdomen full of gas so the pictures they took would be clearer. He was dosed up on painkillers and couldn't be left alone. Neither of us had thought it would be that bad. You hear of people having biopsies all the time, as if it's just a minor procedure with no side effects, but I suppose that's when they're just under the skin, whereas Paul's cysts were internal and they'd had to cut into his abdomen. We were on the start of a very steep learning curve – just because some things are treated as almost everyday medical procedures, it doesn't mean they don't affect the people who have to undergo them, or the people who care for them.

Paul started to feel a little better after a while. He always did feel better when he was at home. He always would. I had already planned to go out that night because I assumed a biopsy was pretty straightforward and that Paul would just get home, have a cup of tea, and be right as rain. I wasn't sure about going, but he insisted I went, telling me it would do me good and he'd probably just doze in front of the telly anyway. So, off I went – to have my fortune told, of all things.

I wasn't a 'believer' – I had just planned to go along with some friends for a laugh. We'd arranged a private session with a psychic and all the girls had questions they wanted to ask. At the back of my mind, though, I did wonder whether this psychic would pick up on what Paul and I had been through that day. If she did, I might be a bit less sceptical about fortune-telling in the future. When I sat down in front of her that evening, she told me a lot of different things – some true, some not – and then she seemed to be referring to Paul when she said it would be OK. One part of me laughed it off – what did she know? – but another bit of me clung gratefully to her words of comfort.

I got home, and Paul was still looking pretty bad. We curled up in bed together and he fell asleep quickly. I lay there, just about to drift off myself. It had been a long and weird day – it certainly seemed like a lifetime ago that we had left the house that morning to go to hospital. Something was niggling at the corner of my consciousness as I tried to drop off. Something I couldn't quite get, couldn't quite catch. Finally, it came to me. As a warning chill ran down my spine, I remembered what the fortune-teller had actually said to me. It wasn't that *Paul* would be OK. It was that *it* would be OK. It would be OK. It would be OK. What did that mean? It hit me immediately exactly what that could mean: things might be OK; I might be OK. I knew that – I knew that I would always be OK, that I could cope with anything. But it didn't necessarily mean that Paul would be OK.

I had a fitful night and went to work at college the next day. I couldn't settle. We had a week to wait for the biopsy results, but it was as if recalling the words of the fortune-teller had opened the floodgates to a reinterpretation of everything else. All morning I thought about the consultant, Mr Sue-Ling, talking about the cysts and I remembered that he had said: 'We need to check if it's a tumour or cysts.' Tumour or cysts. Tumour or cysts. Tumour was a different type of word. Not one you wanted to hear. When I left work and slipped home at lunchtime to look after Paul, I couldn't get the words out of my head.

Alan and Kris were anxious as well. They were going off on holiday and we had to talk them out of cancelling it because they were so worried about Paul's test results. They only went when we promised to let them know as soon as we heard any news.

Over the weekend Paul still couldn't sneeze, cough or laugh without it pulling painfully on his stitches but he still went off to play in the Irish Masters in Dublin. The following days went by in a blur. Paul stayed in Ireland, I went to work. We spoke all the time. I tried to keep things going, tried to focus on what needed to be done rather than letting my mind race away with me.

I wrote in my diary that Wednesday 23 March was D Day. We got up, had breakfast, got dressed and chatted – but never discussed what we were both thinking about: the results. We drove to the hospital and did all the mundane things – parked, checked in at reception, sat in the waiting room, and all the time I kept thinking, PLEASE LET EVERYTHING BE OK. PLEASE LET PAUL BE OK.

Paul walked into the consulting room and I followed. We sat down, went through the usual pleasantries, constantly aware of the folder on the doctor's desk. I tried to read things upside down, tried to read the body language of the consultant. Then the reality hit me. I actually heard what he was saying. In my journal, there are only three words in capital letters:

FUCK. IT'S MALIGNANT.

They had found six tumours. Six. Tumours. I glanced over at Paul and he was as white as a sheet. I couldn't make this better straight away – which is what I always tried to do for him – but I could get information. I went onto autopilot, asking questions, taking notes. I clearly remember the doctor saying that they had also found out that Paul had only one kidney. This seemed to sink in with Paul – he asked all about that, while he didn't really ask about the tumours.

We were told that Paul needed chemotherapy. There were to be three sessions of three days each. Paul would go in on a Wednesday and get his body flushed out with fluid to clean it. The next day at teatime, the chemotherapy would start and chemicals would be drip-fed into his veins all night. The next morning he would get flushed out again and at teatime the next dose of chemo would start. This would be repeated three times, with the idea being to get the chemo in and out of the body as quickly as possible.

What was weird was that I suddenly remembered Paul saying years before that he would get cancer one day. He'd had a few drinks and one of those adverts came on the telly – the ones where they say that one in three people will get cancer – and Paul said, 'That's me. I'm going to be one of the one in three.' I told him not to be so silly, but seemingly he'd repeated this to a few other people who told me about it later. It's strange to think of now. He could be oddly prophetic at times.

Back then, we thought getting cancer was bad luck, for sure, but it was just a question of getting the right treatment and getting cured as soon as possible. But it's not just cancer, is it? It doesn't just come as a lump – there's a whole package of hell to deal with.

And hell was where we were heading.

Chapter Seventeen

Reality

23 March 2005

We drove home in a daze. Quiet. Shocked. Brandon was waiting for us. He was there as much as a friend as anything. We told him all we knew – which wasn't a lot. The doctors had been quite general and said that they needed to do more tests to work out exactly what was going on.

'Are the tumours attached to anything?' asked Brandon. 'Are they attached to any organs?'

Paul looked at him for a moment, then answered: 'Brandon. I have no fucking organs.' He was still focused on the news about only having one kidney. Even though he had lived with that all his life without knowing and without it ever being a problem, it seemed to be the one thing that he fixated on. Maybe it was a distraction.

I cooked Paul a meal and he ate it all. Good sign, I told myself; he's hungry, he's eating. It was surreal. When we had left that morning, everything seemed frightening, but we hadn't been told the dreaded news at that point. It was just the first time the goalposts changed, but that would become a pattern over the next 18 months. To begin with, we had prayed it wouldn't be appendicitis. Later, we would have been happy to take that. Later still, we would have accepted Paul's appendix bursting. That day, we were hoping for cysts. But now, it seemed as if there was nothing left to trade with.

I'd soon find out that you can always sink lower.

When I was alone, I wrote three entries in my journal. I went back to the title page where I had said that I had never felt so happy, that we had no worries, that we were the luckiest of people. Now, above that, I wrote: *Just before our first anniversary … BANG!!!!* Underneath the words about our happiness, I told myself: *We'll get through this, it's just a big stepping stone. Love and strength = positivity.* Inside, I started one of my lists:

Words to hate	*TUMOUR!!!!!!!!!*
	CANCER!!!!!!!!
	MALIGNANT!!!!!!!!
	CHEMOTHERAPY!!!!!!!!
Hate them all.	

I got a text from Paul's mum asking how the test results had been. We decided to lie as they were so far away and couldn't do anything about it. Paul wanted them to enjoy their holiday and not come home early. We told my mum and dad and Tracy that night, though, and they were in shock. What other reaction can you have? Saying the words should make it more real, but they are such awful words that it is hard to make the connection between what they stand for and what they will do to the person you love with all your heart.

That night, when we were alone together, Paul started asking me all the questions he hadn't asked while we were at the hospital. He asked me a lot about chemotherapy but after that he seemed confused and said, 'So, Lindsey – do I have cancer?' How do you answer that? I didn't even want him to ask me in the first place. I took his hands in mine, looked him in the eye and softly said, 'Yes, babes, you do.' He looked like a frightened child. I rubbed his hands in mine and held him as I whispered, 'We'll get rid of the bastard, just you wait and see.' He pulled away and asked, 'Will I lose my hair?' Trust Paul. A life and death battle ahead of him and he was worrying about that. 'Maybe you will, maybe you won't. But you're so gorgeous it won't matter, you'll still look great. Anyway, bandannas suit you, people are used to seeing you in them.'

I didn't just want to comfort him with words. I wished I could take those cysts away from his body and put them in mine. I wanted him to be positive because I was convinced it would help, but he didn't seem to be thinking that way. Paul's mum phoned, obviously not entirely convinced by our earlier text. 'Are you sure you're telling us everything?' she asked. 'What exactly did the doctor say?' But Paul was adamant that she shouldn't be told at this stage. I'm not so sure she believed us when we said that the tests were inconclusive and that Paul would need to go back for more of the same. But the words were easy to say, they made it seem for a moment as if it wasn't happening.

* * *

I didn't sleep that night.

The next day when I went to work, everyone asked about the test results. I wished I'd never mentioned them in the first place but we had genuinely thought it was just a problem with Paul's appendix so we were completely open about it. I had to stop these conversations dead so I told them that we had to wait another two weeks for the results. It was a lie but I couldn't talk about the truth yet.

Paul was interviewed by a journalist that day and they also asked him about the 'cysts' (goodness knows how they had heard). He was fantastic, just coming out with the same line about having to wait a bit longer. I was so proud of him but in private I broke down and had a really good cry.

Two days later, on 26 March, Paul was due to fly to China for a big event. Since he was now so popular out there, he had been asked to go a bit early to do publicity. He decided that he would still travel, so he flew off and I was left alone to think about it all without him there. I tried to keep myself busy and practical as always, but when I read what I wrote in my diary, I wonder to what extent I was hoping for a miracle: *Maybe it will all go away if he's in another country ...*

One of the ways I've coped through all of this – to this day – is by sectioning things off. You can't be miserable all of the time. It's just not possible to get on with living your life that way. I have good memories and I have bad memories. We all do. The way I deal with them is to have doors in my mind, or little boxes. I put the bad things in the boxes or behind the doors and shut them away. I take them out again when I'm ready to deal with them, but I don't let them run riot. They're not allowed out all the time. It's not that I'm never sad, that I never cry; it's just that I try to control it. I put happy memories away too. I have a door behind which is Paul's first visit to the clinic when they talked about chemo – but I also have one where Paul is waiting to pick me up in his car for the first time ever back in March 1997. I have one where his hair has all fallen out and he looks grey – but I also have one where I've just given birth and we are holding our baby daughter together.

Going back to think about that first day we knew about the cancer is very hard. I can smell the hospital, I can see the peeling wallpaper in my mind's eye. I can relive the way Paul wasn't taking much in, apart from the news about his kidney. And I remember how he seemed to think I knew best, so when I said, 'Be positive, get through chemo, then you'll be fine,' he believed it.

So did I at the time.

Chapter Eighteen

'Your husband's got cancer'

March 2005

While Paul was in China, we spoke constantly – in fact, by the end of the trip, his mobile phone bill was over £1,000. The first Sunday he was there, I went round to my mum's for lunch and Paul rang while I was there. Not only was he a bit drunk, he was also inconsolable. The tears were really flowing by the time he called; I think it had all just started to hit him. God, it was awful – what can you do when you're so far apart? He couldn't stop crying, and I couldn't help but think that the tears would do him some good, perhaps help him to accept what was going on and prepare himself for the fight. He was on a mission to get wasted, I wrote in my diary, and I couldn't really blame him. What I didn't know was what was really happening in China.

He had told Jimmy White almost as soon as they arrived. Jimmy had got through testicular cancer in the past and Paul thought a great deal of him, so it was natural that he would be the first fellow snooker player that Paul would confide in. According to another player, Jimmy Michie, for the first time ever, Paul wasn't the affable bloke they had all relied on. He was upset. He was almost hysterical. Jimmy says he even broke one of his own rules by going round telling certain people that he'd never liked them. That was so out of character that it must have shocked the people close to him more than anything.

I wasn't being let off lightly either. He must have rung about 15 times in succession that Sunday and with every call he was getting drunker and nastier. I went back to the house and stayed there for the night, because Paul had told me he didn't want me going out, and I just took one call after another. His pain and anger poured out. He called me lots of horrible names, but I knew he wouldn't remember in the morning. It didn't matter to me – I knew he was just getting things out of his system. It's human nature to kick out at the ones you love the most; they are the ones you know won't hold a grudge. I let him vent all his anger; I just wanted to hold him and tell him it would be all right.

He kept pushing me to say, 'My husband has cancer.' He was screaming at me: 'Say it! Fucking say it!' I wouldn't, so he got angrier and angrier, more and more names were hurled at me, and he kept shouting, 'Your husband's got cancer! Fucking say it, Lindsey! Your husband's got cancer!' Eventually he wore himself out and the calls stopped – his heart was breaking. I could tell that, no matter how far away we were from each other.

I stumbled through the next few days, trying to keep normal life going. Paul was still in China, and amazingly on the Wednesday he won his match. That made him feel better and gave him a bit of a positive lift. The day after that, he played Jimmy White, and from Paul being 4–0 up, Jimmy managed to pull it back to 4–3. That would please Paul in lots of ways – not only was he back to being himself at the table (going to the brink of losing), but it also showed that Jimmy wasn't treating him any differently since he knew about the cancer. It must have given Paul a boost because he eventually won the match 5–3. I wrote in my diary: *Our luck is changing.* I genuinely felt that way. Snooker was so important to Paul; it gave him a foundation. I felt that any positive news would help, whether it came from snooker wins or anything else.

The next day, however, Paul lost to Ken Doherty 5–1. He didn't get many chances in the match, but the good side was that he was on his way home. After a seven-hour wait in Frankfurt, Paul was due back on Saturday night at 9.30pm just over a week since he had left. It was wonderful to see him, but an hour after he got off the flight, his luggage still hadn't turned up. His case was one thing – you can always replace clothes – but his snooker cue was missing as well. With the World Championship coming up in only two weeks' time, this was something else for Paul to worry about. It probably seems insignificant to anyone else, but a player's cue means so much to them; Paul always felt that his cue held lots of his past history, the magic of his wins. By Sunday lunchtime, when there was still no sign, he was frantic. When it finally turned up later that day, we both felt so relieved – as if it mattered.

* * *

Paul had no sooner got over that problem than his next hurdle appeared. His mum and dad were coming to our house and they would have to be told. I urged Paul to try not to make it sound too bad; I wanted to protect him and I was scared that Kristina and Alan might fall to bits and that, in turn, would have a negative effect on him. What was I thinking? Now that I have Evie Rose, I can't imagine how anyone can tell you that your child has tumours and make it sound anything less than horrendous.

We both felt sick waiting for them to arrive. At 3pm, the doorbell rang. I tried to keep things normal at first, as if that would cushion the news. We stalled for a while, showing them our new sofa and the bathroom that we'd just finished off, then I gave Paul 'the look' as if to nudge him, 'Say it now.' Even now, I can remember that he had this weird smile on his face – it was as if he was smirking before he opened his mouth. It worried me but I guess it was just a nervous reaction. He started to talk and I butted in, worried about how he was going to present it to his mum and dad. I tried to keep it clear and logical even though my head was spinning.

'What do you mean – tumours?' Kris asked. 'What kind of tumours? What are they going to do about them?'

Alan looked sick. 'He's only young. It can't be anything serious. The doctors will sort it out, won't they?'

We told them about the type of treatments that were available, then Paul told them that he had an appointment that Wednesday, 6th April, at 10.30am with Dr Gilby, and it was decided that we would all go, in force, united, ready to fight – ready to fight for Paul.

At one point when Paul wasn't listening, I whispered to them: 'Please keep the tears for when you're at home, with someone else, anywhere but in front of him.' Kris didn't cry in front of Paul at all and I was grateful for that. I think Alan went to the bathroom and had a cry there. When they finally left that night, they went to see Paul's Auntie Teresa and cousin Anthony. Then they had to say the dreaded words themselves – 'Paul's got cancer' – and it was at that point that Kristina says she broke down.

Chapter Nineteen

Dread

6 April 2005

We got through the next few days on autopilot. We knew Paul had to go into battle, but we had no idea of exactly what was ahead. I kept up my positive attitude as much as I could. I spent the Monday with Paul's sister, Leanne, and we spoke about her forthcoming wedding and all sorts of 'normal' things. On the Tuesday, I told close work colleagues what was happening. Every time the conversation veered around to Paul, I'd just make myself all jolly again. 'It'll be fine; we'll be fine; everything will be fine.' Did I believe it myself? I probably did at that point, but it didn't stop me writing in my diary that I was dreading Wednesday and that all I could really do was keep my fingers crossed.

Wednesday 6 April took forever to come, and, at the same time, it came far too soon. We both woke up feeling lousy and somehow managed to arrive at St. James' Hospital almost two hours ahead of Paul's appointment. I was so glad Kris and Alan were there with us that day because they were both really strong and supportive. The specialist we saw was a Dr Anthoney (we had been referred to him by Dr Gilby), someone who would be there for a lot of Paul's hospital visits and treatments. He got straight to the point.

'Paul,' he began, 'I have to be honest with you. I'm still not 100 per cent sure what type of cancer we're dealing with here. It may be testicular, it may be a neuro-endocrine tumour. We have to look at lots of possibilities. What I would like to do is show you the images we got during your laparoscopy, when we found six cysts.'

When he showed Paul the films, it looked more like two hundred than six. I couldn't get the image out of my head and neither could Paul, who later said that he wished he hadn't seen it as it made him feel sick knowing what was inside his body. Perhaps there were only six technically, but they looked the way chocolate Maltesers look when they melt and stick together. It was as if they had all welded into what looked to us like huge masses of disgusting lumps. They weren't attached to organs but were clumped inside the abdominal cavity. I asked if they couldn't just operate and cut them out but they said no, that wasn't possible.

Paul was taken for an ultrasound on his testicles, but there were no tumours showing there. I sat waiting for almost an hour and a half trying to convince myself that hospitals weren't so bad. I was going to have to get used to them, so I'd better start believing it. I tried to focus on things that were real – the colour of the walls, the people sitting beside me – just to keep my mind away from what was happening to Paul. When I saw someone standing outside the hospital

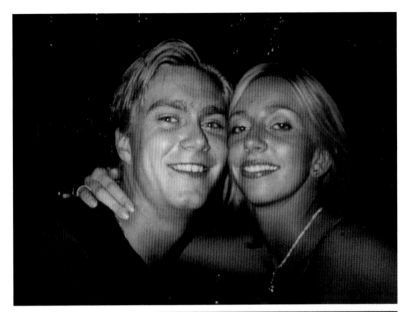

Above The Banyon Tree, Thailand in 2002. One of many fantastic holidays Paul and I had together.

Right The Benson & Hedges Masters, 2002. Paul was only the third player in the history of the tournament to defend his Masters' title successfully, winning it for a second time here.

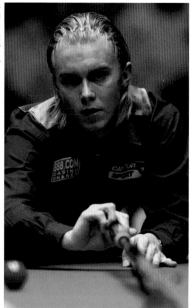

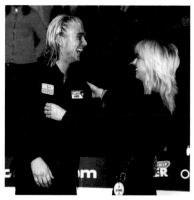

Above The tension was over. He'd done it again and won the 'battle of the popstars', beating Ronnie O'Sullivan in the 2004 Masters final. It was Paul's third Masters' title in four years.

Above Here's my cool, confident Paul in the zone.

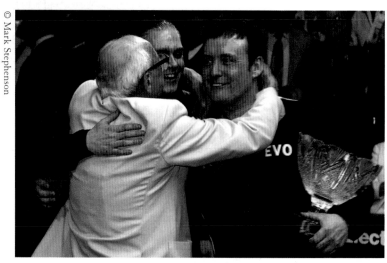

Paul hugs Jimmy White and Jimmy's dad, Tommy, after losing the 2004 Daily Record Players Championship. A result which cost Paul £70,000. Look at Paul's face – he could lose with as much grace as when he was a winner.

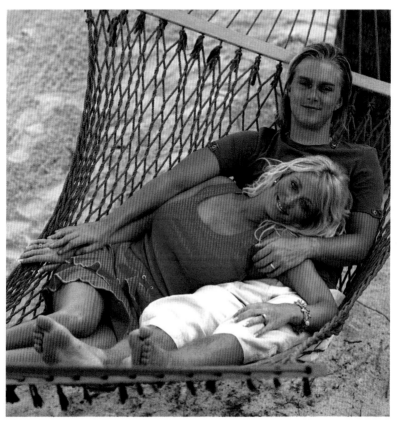

Above Our honeymoon, on Negril Beach, Jamaica, in May 2004. I love this picture of Paul. He was so gorgeous. I was so proud.

Left Our wedding day – 19th May 2004. On the cliff at Rick's Café, Jamaica, during the evening ceremony. By that time, we had all become a little merry and everyone was laying bets on whether we'd fall off the cliff into the sea!

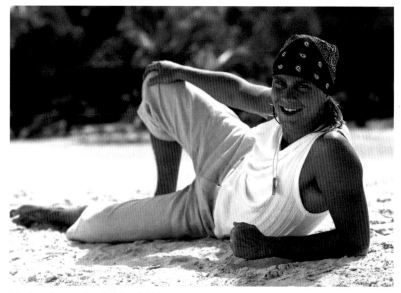

My handsome Paul, May 2004.

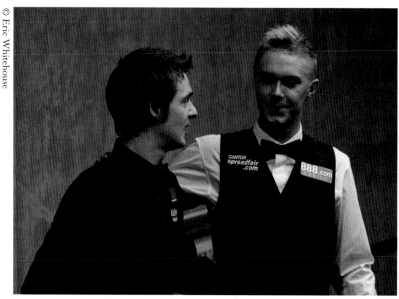

The World Championships, 2005. This was when Paul announced to the world that he had cancer. Having lost the match to Michael Holt (here), now he was facing the biggest fight of his life.

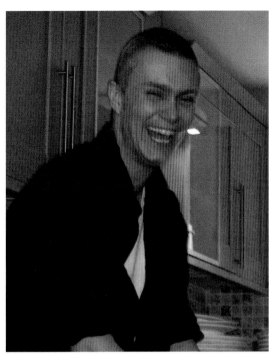

Left March 2006. Paul on alternative medicine – the 'loony juice'. He was happy not to be on chemo any more.

Below Paul and me with our beautiful Evie Rose. At this point, we were both afraid of what the future would hold for us.

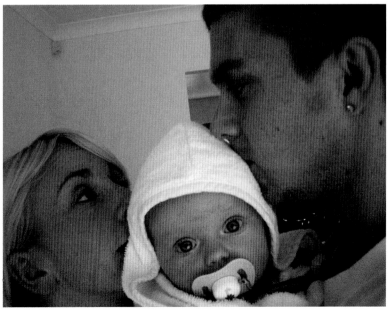

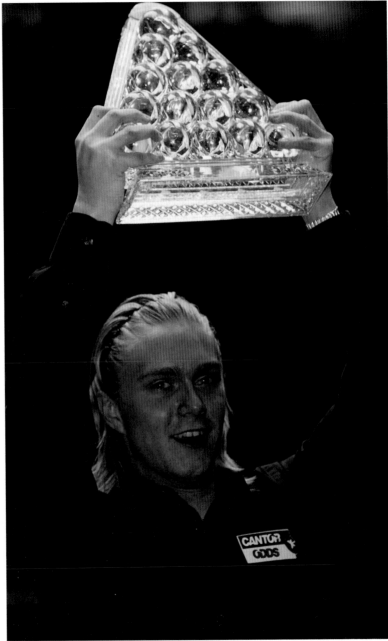

2004 Masters. This is how we will all remember Paul. A champion of life.

entrance with a drip in one hand and a cigarette in the other, it made me feel physically ill.

At 12.30pm, we were taken in to see another specialist, Dr Chester, and a member of the support team, Carolyn Cook. There was a bit of general talk, but it was clear to me that their aim was to get Paul to say things out loud, and, presumably accept them into the bargain.

I remember Dr Chester asking him, 'What do you think you've got, Paul?'

Paul looked at him stony-faced. 'I've got cancer.'

'What type of cancer do you think you've got, Paul?'

'A rare type. Well, it stands to reason – I'm unique, aren't I?'

If this was meant to make Paul break down in some way, it wasn't going to work. The doctor talked about chemotherapy and how often Paul would have to have it, and Paul responded by asking if he could wait until after the World Snooker Championship, due to start in the next couple of weeks. As he wasn't showing any symptoms yet, it was agreed that it would be fine for him to delay chemo. Was this the right decision? I don't know – there were lots of things we were in the dark about back then, huge areas of knowledge I didn't yet have. As I wrote in my diary that night:

God, they're giving him a real blast of chemo. This is going to be tough. It's funny the world we live in. No one asks the important question – 'Am I going to die?' Paul was more worried about whether he was going to lose his hair. I don't suppose they have that many lads in there with long blond ponytails, but still … there were other things to be asked.

Dr Chester and Carolyn told Paul about the risk of infections, and the loss of sensation he might experience in his fingertips, as well as dozens of other things. I got the impression that they would pretty much take him to the edge of death before bringing him back again.

Paul had 15 blood samples taken that day and he was so brave and positive. He didn't like the sound of checks for HIV, AIDS and syphilis – I think he took that as a personal slight – but they reassured him it was common practice for everyone. The four of us went for lunch, hardly able to believe that it was only half an hour since the meeting with Dr Chester. He'd told us so much that we'd only taken in a fraction of it. I admit that I did have a little cry at that point to relieve some of the pressure; and I felt better after it. Paul was concentrating on other things, pointing out that we wouldn't be able to go to Cyprus for his sister's wedding in July. It was disappointing, but we were fast realizing that there are some issues that matter in the grand scheme of things and some that really don't.

It was non-stop for the rest of the day. We went back to get Paul's appointment times for the coming weeks. All the staff were so nice, as if he was the only patient there. How do people deal with that sort of job, knowing that every day of work will bring another heartbreaking story?

The doctors said that they were 'treating it to cure it'. I decided to hang onto those words and repeat them every day. They raised the issue of Paul's fertility – chemotherapy can affect a man's sperm count, but it's also advised that you avoid trying to become pregnant during treatment as no one is quite sure how it might affect the foetus. The doctor said that Paul would be able to make a deposit in a sperm bank and decide whether to go down that route at a later date. Paul still managed to make me laugh. When he was given an appointment to do this at 2pm the following Monday, he said, 'Well, that's the easy part of everything – how difficult can having a wank be?'

It was decision after decision, appointment after appointment. We got home about 3.45pm and my head was buzzing but Paul seemed quite calm. Kris and Alan left, having held themselves together all day, but I suspected they might break down when they got home.

Brandon phoned to ask what we wanted to do about the press. People knew Paul hadn't been well and the appendicitis story had been doing the rounds. However, he had told a few snooker players and his behaviour in China wouldn't have gone unnoticed. On top of that, even though it was horrible to think about, we were warned that there could be leaks from the staff at the hospital. Paul wanted to be straightforward and honest about it all, so Brandon released a press statement (which is often misinterpreted to this day as saying Paul had stomach cancer), and within 10 minutes it was everywhere. It was on Sky text, it was on the TV news, and the next morning it was in all the papers. Everybody seemed to know within seconds. The texts came flooding in and the phones wouldn't stop ringing.

And what was Paul doing in the middle of all this? He was outside filling a skip with rubbish from the bathroom makeover. I thought he was amazing. He had never once asked 'why me?' But I also knew that it would be a different matter once he had a drink inside him, which always made him emotional.

It only took another day. On the Thursday he decided to get hammered with his mates, Bear and Naeem. I asked him to stay at home because I knew the tears wouldn't take long to come – and I was right. He woke me after midnight in floods.

'Lindsey, I think I'm going to die,' he cried. 'I'm so, so scared. I don't know what to do. God, I wouldn't wish this on anyone. Help me, Lindsey, help me, please. I don't want to die, I don't want to die.' It went on for a while, but it cleared the tension a bit by the time he got himself under control.

I told him there and then, 'Paul – alcohol is NO good for positive thinking. If you're going to drink, you're going to have to accept that it'll have this effect on you.' He was full of promises, but I knew he wouldn't keep them. What I didn't know was that there would come a time when I'd be the one desperate for him to have a drink and escape from himself for at least a little while.

Things seemed a little better the next day. Everyone knew, thanks to Brandon's press release, and Paul decided to go to an exhibition match in Morley. I was glad. All the people there were lovely to him, and he was an absolute saint. He played very well and there was no sign of tears. We both felt genuinely happy that night, and so pleased that we had had a good day to balance out the one before.

As we fell into each other's arms that night, we had no

idea just how good a day it was really going to be. This would be the last time we were allowed to have sex before Paul made his 'deposit'. As we giggled together about the sperm bank visit on Monday, neither of us knew that Evie Rose had decided it was time for her to make an appearance. Any visits to the sperm bank would turn out to be unnecessary because, after several months of trying, I conceived that night, just two days after we had stared death in the face for the first time.

Chapter Twenty

Life goes on

11 April 2005

*P*aul played more exhibition matches over the weekend and did well, with two excellent breaks of 136 and 135. Professionally, he seemed to be able to remain totally focused despite what was going on in his personal life. As Monday came, he was still joking about the visit to the sperm bank and saying this was one appointment at Jimmy's that he was looking forward to. I wasn't looking forward to Monday, though; I was feeling sick at the thought of Paul's HIV and STD tests coming back. I knew he hadn't always been an angel before we settled down, but I didn't think I could cope with some piece of paper pointing it out to me. And chances are if he had something, I would have it as well. We needed to be strong together for what was ahead, not split by angry memories of things in the past.

We arrived half an hour early and waited 90 minutes to see someone. I was red hot with worry and my chest was all blotchy to prove it. Paul signed consent form after consent form then the results arrived. I held my breath until he said, 'It's clear!'

The Assisted Conception Unit at St James' gave the next procedure a completely clinical description: we were there 'for the purpose of pre-chemotherapy sperm banking as the proposed treatment could affect your ability to produce sperm and affect your future fertility.' There were lots of guidelines to consider, regulations of the Human Fertilization and Embryology Act, ethical implications, obligations and counselling options. All I thought was that Paul might not be able to father a baby for a long time, perhaps never, after his chemo – and we desperately wanted one. We had been trying for what seemed ages, but I still hadn't got pregnant (as far as I knew then). There were plenty of times when we weren't even in the same country, never mind the same bed, at the part of my cycle when we should have been trying.

Paul was given a little pot for his sample. Off he trotted, and 10 minutes later arrived back with the same pot in his pocket with not very much in it. He handed it to the nurse and it took two hours to get checked for sperm count and motility. I asked him why there wasn't much and he sheepishly admitted that his aim wasn't quite right and most of it missed the pot. It broke the atmosphere as we joked about our future kids lying on the floor of a hospital room waiting to get mopped up. There was a part of me that wondered whether I was being selfish, still pushing for a baby when Paul didn't even know what lay ahead of him – but he wanted a little one just as much as I did and it was good to have something positive in the future to look forward to.

As all of that went on, as we laughed, neither Paul nor I

had any notion of the flurry of test results that were being analysed, and the many notes being sent between one department and another about the findings.

To us, Paul had been in pain and we had suspected appendicitis but had been told cancer. This wasn't how the doctors put it. Their diagnosis was very detailed and depressing-sounding:

METASTATIC INTRA-ABDOMINAL CARCINOMA – MOST LIKELY NEUROENDOCRINE CARCINOMA WITH GERM CELL DIFFERENTIATION ALTHOUGH POSSIBLY SERTOLI CELL TUMOUR OR GERM CELL TUMOUR WITH NEUROENDOCRINE DIFFERENTIATION

Now that I have some of Paul's records (and it was hard work getting those), it's not just the medical terms that seem confusing; it's the fact that they seem much more negative than Paul and I thought at the time. From that first appointment onwards, we clung to any positive words the doctors used. However, the notes from the specialist in the Germ Cell Clinic addressed to the staff at the Neuro-endocrine Clinic are much more gloomy from the outset: 'Whilst we cannot be entirely certain what this unusual tumour is, it is most likely to represent a neuro-endocrine tumour, *of a relatively poor prognostic type ... the prognosis is unlikely to be nearly as good as for testicular cancer.*' (My italics.)

They go on: 'Paul and his family seem to understand the issues and be remarkably calm about the situation. He was not keen to talk statistics and survival times, so I have left those discussions for another occasion, but he is aware that this is unlikely to be as curable as a testicular cancer.'

I remember Paul being confused when the doctor explained to him that it would be better if it was testicular cancer. 'I don't want cancer of the bloody bollocks!' he'd exclaimed, with a typical male reaction. I think we were overwhelmed by the terms used, and very alarmed that they didn't seem clear about the diagnosis. Certainly neither of us picked up that the prognosis was poor from the start. We just wanted them to find out what it was, and tell us what cure to take.

Everything kept changing. We had prayed that it wasn't his appendix and ended up wishing it was. Now, we had to recognize that when we had prayed it wouldn't be testicular cancer, that's what we should have been hoping for. Everything was topsy turvy, but life had to go on.

I went back into work at college the day after the sperm bank deposit, and the day after that we were back at Jimmy's for kidney tests. It's amazing how quickly things become normalized – in my diary I've written: *Today went well, 9.30am injection of radium.* Whatever happened to my diary being all about our blissful newlyweds' life?

I was starting to learn all sorts of medical terminology. I learned that germ cell tumours tended to develop from sperm cells (or egg cells in women) and were easier to treat than neuro-endocrine tumours that developed from nerve cells. I also learned that alpha feta protein (AFP) blood tests are used to detect certain kinds of cancers. The higher the score, the bigger the tumour. AFP levels should get back down to normal after chemotherapy but if they don't, that means the tumour hasn't completely gone. At this point, Paul's AFP tumour markers were 19,000, up from 12,000. In a healthy, non-cancerous person, the level is tiny, somewhere between 0 and 5 for most, going up even to 30 in some. We would become obsessed by these figures. Every time Paul had a blood test, we'd wait for the tumour marker level result and it became the guide as to whether we should be celebrating or not.

The day after the kidney tests, Paul went to the Premier League tournament and had an amazing reception. Every time he spoke about his fight with cancer, everyone started chanting his name. I was nearly in tears. It sounds daft I know, but I was also thinking that this was the last time for a while that Paul would have his trademark long hair. He was due to get it cut the next day, in preparation for chemo, and while I know that in the grand scheme of things it didn't matter at all, it still upset me. I could hardly believe that it was less than a year ago when I had seen him go off on his stag night worrying that the lads would shave his head. A year ago but a world away.

When we woke up next morning, I thought I'd never seen his hair look so beautiful. It was shining, golden – full of life. I think I was more nervous than him. Maybe there is a part of you that feels it's wrong to be cutting something healthy; maybe it feels like tempting fate. Paul wasn't bothered in the slightest and wanted to get it cut in some outrageous style but I talked him out of that, and I took some pictures as his first locks fell. After it was all over, he looked even better than before. Not Brad Pitt or David Beckham or any of the other heart-throbs he was always being compared to – this was all Paul Hunter and he was more gorgeous than ever.

The next day he went off to Sheffield for the 2005 World Championships, keen to show off his new hairstyle and the two diamond stud earrings he was going to flaunt to the world.

I couldn't get there until the following day as I had to do an interview on telly with Hazel Irvine, the *Grandstand* presenter. She wanted to talk about how we were coping, what type of cancer Paul was fighting, what the outcome was likely to be, and all that sort of thing. God, I was nervous! These days doing telly doesn't bother me at all, but that day my lips kept sticking to my gums and my red, patchy chest was out in force.

When the first match started, the announcer said: 'I know you'll have your own special welcome for the boy with the golden cue,' and the crowd went crazy. I was close to tears and Paul must have felt it too, even though he held himself together very well. If only we could have bottled all that love and goodwill and support. I was so proud of him.

Of course, in a fairy story, Paul would battle through the World Championship and win. Real life isn't like that though – he lost 10–8 in his first match. It was so close, and he had clawed his way back from behind plenty of times before, but who knows what effect the last few weeks had had on him? Who knows how he even managed to get out there and play at all?

It was very emotional for Paul, leaving the hall to a standing ovation and wondering when he would be back there again and what he would have to go through first. He had just got into his dressing room with Brandon when suddenly there was a knock on the door. Two guys in blazers were standing there and they announced that Paul had been randomly selected to do a drugs test. All finalists are tested at every tournament and a small number of participants' names are pulled out of a hat as well.

Brandon was furious. 'Have you got any idea what this kid's going through?' he asked them. 'Do you have any human sympathy?'

He shut the door and went in to discuss it with Paul. There were two problems about doing the test. First of all, they didn't know what drugs the doctors at Jimmy's had been giving him to test whether his body was ready for the chemo. But secondly, Paul was emotionally strung out and just wanted to get home. If he did the test, he'd have to hang around drinking loads of fluid until he could fill their two big sample bottles with urine. They decided he wasn't going to do it and Brandon went back out to tell the officials his decision.

The tournament director was there, and Brandon rebuked him: 'Couldn't you just have overlooked it when his name was pulled out? Would that have been too much to ask?'

For some people, rules are rules though. A month later, in

the middle of his chemo, Paul was sent a letter from the World Snooker Association with documentation from UK Sport outlining the potential disciplinary action he could face in due course for not taking the drugs test. The World Snooker governing body let Paul down that day and didn't find a way to support him during his illness; they didn't seem to have a safety net for players who were suffering from any form of illness. It took a full three months for the governing body to decide there would be no further action on the matter.

As he left Sheffield that day in April 2005, everyone gathered round to wish him well. He could hardly get out of the place for fans wanting to shake his hand and pat him on the back. I didn't want to leave. I knew that as soon as we got home, the fight would really commence.

Chapter Twenty-one

The battle begins

19 April 2005

We woke up on Tuesday 19 April to a beautiful sunny day. Things didn't seem too bad as we drove to Cookridge Hospital for Paul to have a brain and body scan. He sipped an aniseed drink for 45 minutes and then off he went. I sat there trying to find hospitals less threatening than I used to. I was thinking that the weather was beautiful, the people at hospital were friendly, but really I was hanging on by a thread.

When Paul came out, I asked him 'How was it, babes?' He looked straight at me before replying, 'It was awful. It was awful. Losing 10–8 is nothing compared to lying having a brain scan to see if the cancer has spread there too.'

The mood changed like that. On a finger snap. I still thought that we had to stay positive, but how could I keep saying that to him when he was the one going through such horrible experiences? We popped over to get the results of the sperm tests – the count was a bit low but, in general, everything in that department was good.

We made our way home and Paul was very quiet. Later that night, my friend Sally came over and we got roaring drunk, which left me feeling extremely sick in the morning. Really unwell. I suppose it was my way of dealing with the pressure. Maybe it was better to be a little bit anaesthetized by a hangover because we had quite a day ahead of us.

As soon as we got through the hospital doors, I started my usual silent mantra: 'Please, please, please let it be good news.' Suddenly, I realized what I was saying and that there was no way it could be 'good', so I changed my words to: 'Please, please, please let it be goodish news.' I didn't think Paul could take any more at this stage.

There are certain things you never want to hold in your hand or be in possession of. An appointment card for a Medical Oncology Department is one of those. For me, another was the blue ring binder which contained 'all you need to know about chemotherapy'. It's one of those words that people use almost carelessly – they'll talk about a friend or a work colleague or a family member having chemo, and everyone just nods and thinks they know what it's all about.

Unless you've been there, you have no idea.

The blue folder went over the bare bones of what was facing Paul.

Chemotherapy is treatment with drugs which destroy or control cancer cells. Chemotherapy drugs stop cancer cells from growing and spreading. The cancer cells become damaged and eventually die. We will usually give you chemotherapy as several courses of treatment so it can kill as many cancer cells as possible. Unfortunately, chemotherapy drugs can affect normal cells in your body as well, and this sometimes causes unpleasant side effects. However, normal cells regrow and heal quickly so the damage is only temporary. Most side effects disappear completely when the treatment is over.

We would cling onto lots of those words once treatment started: 'stop cancer cells from growing'; 'cancer cells become damaged'; 'normal cells regrow'. We were given a fact sheet about the chemotherapy regime Paul was to be treated with – its full name was Bleomycin/Etoposide/Cisplatin, or BEP. A powder was dissolved in liquid to make a clear fluid that was drip-fed through a cannula into Paul's vein. The list of potential side effects was lengthy and, even though we were told they probably wouldn't *all* affect Paul, we were also told that there could be others, rarer ones, that he might suffer from. The list was horrendous but the most common were:

Temporary reduction in bone marrow function
Anaemia
Unexplained bruising or bleeding
Nausea and vomiting
Kidney problems
Hair loss including eyelashes, eyebrows and other body hair
Fever and chills
Skin changes including rash, excess pigment production
Mouth sores and ulcers

Changes in nails
Changes to the lungs
Numbness or tingling in the hands or feet
Changes in hearing
Loss of appetite / temporary taste alterations
Fertility
Diarrhoea
Allergic reactions
Sensitivity of the skin to sunlight

We didn't know at the outset, but Paul was going to get most of them.

He was given a list of contact numbers – a 24-hour emergency number; ward number; outpatient clinic; research nurse; intravenous team; oncology specialist nurse; transport; switchboard. That folder and those leaflets made it perfectly clear that this wasn't going to be a walk in the park.

I think, to some extent, we're almost used to cancer these days. It's much less common than it used to be to hear of young people getting it and you read all the time that it can be beaten, that chemotherapy is incredible, that a positive diagnosis isn't a death sentence. We remembered all of that – and believed it. We had to.

The outpatients department was running an hour late – we didn't know yet that this was par for the course. Paul's doctor was delayed because he was discussing the scan with another consultant. Why? What were they discussing? Had it spread? Had something happened? As all this was going through my mind – and no doubt through Paul's too –

Carolyn was telling him how good his new haircut looked. We all laughed and chatted as if it was the most natural place to be in the world. This was something we'd both have to get used to. Any tiny little bit of normality – like a new haircut – was grabbed with force and every last bit of chat wrung out of it, while no one ever talked about the fact that it was necessary in the first place because some evil disease was coursing through the body of the man you love, threatening everything you have.

We sat in the waiting room moaning about delays and wishing everyone would hurry up – then, as soon as we walked towards the consulting room, our stomachs tensed up. I wanted to drag Paul away and protect him with my love. If they didn't say bad things, maybe everything would be all right.

It turned out that Paul's tumour markers were up to 20,000 but the cancer didn't seem to have spread anywhere else. The doctor said that Paul was doing really well and that it was a good idea to start chemotherapy the following week, as planned. Paul was given lots of information – how many visitors he could have and when, what food he should eat, and several things we didn't know about, like a device called a cold cap that patients can wear to try and prevent hair loss.

The doctor talked about the BEP chemotherapy still being the best option, but also raised the fact that experts in London had suggested introducing a drug called Streptozocin into the treatment. He said he still thought that BEP was the best way forward at this point. I felt a bit uneasy when there were different options mentioned – I wanted there to be one straight path, one straight cure for Paul.

He had more blood taken and was told that his single kidney was working well. Mostly, it was me who asked the questions and took things in, but at one point, Paul spoke: 'This treatment,' he said. 'Will it shrink the cancer? Will the tumour go away?'

The doctor wasn't evasive – he didn't have a crystal ball but he was used to percentages, to odds. 'If this was a germ cell tumour, Paul,' he said, 'the chance of the tumour shrinking would be very high, probably around 75–80 per cent. If, on the other hand, this is not a germ cell tumour, the chance of objective response is around one in three.' It felt like we were back at square one – back to wishing for one awful thing instead of another; now we were being told that some tumours are better than others. 'See you next Tuesday,' the consultant called as we left the room.

Next Tuesday.

As if it were the most ordinary thing in the world.

Next Tuesday, my Paul was going to start chemotherapy. It had to work. It just had to.

Chapter Twenty-two

A ray of hope

24 April 2005

I didn't heed my own warning about too much drink bringing out the tears. Two days after the clinic visit, Paul went on a boy's night out (it actually started in the afternoon), that he referred to as 'The Last Supper'. The girls went out for a meal and then we all met up around half past ten. Everyone was completely smashed and, after two hours, when people were starting to drift home, the mood changed. To start with it had been noisy and fun, but then friends started to be too nice and gave us 'that look', which showed how sorry they were feeling for us. Paul wanted to go once that happened but people were holding onto him, crying. Those who weren't sobbing their hearts out were too wrecked to stand, or stuck in the loo being ill.

The pair of us managed to get away but the emotion was affecting us too. We slumped in the corner of our bedroom in tears, and cried our eyes out for hours, until 4.30am. Through the tears, Paul sobbed: 'Everyone thinks I'm strong, Linz, but I'm not. I'm not. I'm scared.'

It was hard to comfort him when I was in pieces too, but I tried. 'People know it's hard, Paul – they know it's one of the hardest things in the world. They know it isn't easy and probably just think you're putting on a brave face. It's OK to cry sometimes, babes, but you do have to keep strong, you do have to keep positive, we *will* fight this and we *will* win.' I held onto him as tightly as I could, but our hearts were breaking. The next day I went into work absolutely knackered. I'd had a fair bit to drink, we all had, but this was worse than my usual hangovers. I felt sick and exhausted and, to top it all, my period was due – in fact it was already a day late, so I'd have that to cope with as well when it came.

I don't know how I got through the day but somehow I staggered on. As I checked over the following week's appointments in my diary, I noticed that I'd made a mistake. I wasn't a day late; I was three days late – and that never happens to me. I'm regular as clockwork. I could hardly let myself even think it but ... could I be pregnant?

When I got home that night, Paul and I just watched telly. I sat on the sofa with him and thought, 'This is all I've ever wanted. To curl up on the sofa with the man I love watching Saturday night telly.' It didn't seem much to ask, but I knew that there had been moments in the past few weeks when even this ordinariness had seemed unattainable. We'd had to learn pretty quickly to put hospitals and cancer and tests and chemo out of our minds whenever we could; it would eat away at everything given half a chance.

As we lay there, my mind kept flickering to the dates in my diary. Wouldn't I know if I was pregnant? I had felt a bit sick, but I had been drinking quite a bit too. Oh God! If I *was* pregnant, would the baby be damaged by my alcohol intake? One second, I was thinking along those lines, then the next I'd hear a little voice saying, 'Don't be stupid, Lindsey – you've been trying to get pregnant for months and months at a time when Paul was perfectly healthy. Do you really think that days after he was diagnosed, two days before he begins chemotherapy, it would suddenly have worked?'

It was hard to keep it from Paul, but I didn't want him to get his hopes up only to dash them. The next morning Paul woke up desperate for a bacon sandwich. I had a quick shower, grabbed some clothes, and drove to Asda – the perfect excuse to go out and get a pregnancy test. I came back, made Paul a sarnie and then headed to the loo. I checked the instructions about a dozen times, and each time I realized it was just as simple as it had seemed on first reading. Take stick out of wrapper. Take lid off. Pee on stick. Wait. Check result. No hidden difficulties, no way I could get it wrong.

Two minutes to wait.

Longest two minutes ever.

Check the result.

Check the result again.

Check it again and again and again.

I thought there had to be a mistake – because it was telling me that it was positive, that I was pregnant! I'd rehearsed this moment in my mind over and over again. Now that it was finally here, all I could do was bolt down the stairs and shove the stick at Paul. He was completely non-plussed. I couldn't believe there was no reaction.

'Paul!' I shrieked. 'Well? What do you think?'

'What's this?' he asked, glancing at the stick. 'What do I do with it? What's it for?'

It dawned on me that, after so many tests, he thought this was another one for him. He thought it was something else from the hospital!

'Paul,' I said, 'it's not a test for you; it's a test for me.'

He looked at me blankly. 'What are you getting tested for?'

'It's my test, Paul. I'm testing to see if I'm pregnant, babes. And I am!'

'NO!' he shouted. 'NO! You're not pregnant? Are you pregnant Linz? Are you? Really?'

He looked at the cigarette in his hand and said, 'God, I need to put that out,' but he couldn't – his hand was shaking too much. Neither of us really believed what we were seeing.

My first thought was that if someone would know for sure, it would be Tracy, since she had two kids already. When we arrived, she and her husband took ages showing us round bits of the house they'd been doing up, but we finally sat down in the conservatory. I didn't say anything, just handed the stick to my big sister.

Her reaction was immediate – and loud. 'I can't believe it! I can't believe it, Linz!'

'D'you think it's right then, our Trace?' I asked her.

'Of course it's right! They're hardly ever wrong. Oh, Lindsey, this is the best news ever. This is what will get us through Paul's treatment,' she said, hugging us both.

It was just what I had been thinking too. This could be

our lucky charm, the ray of light that would make the darkness bearable. God, I hoped nothing would go wrong with the pregnancy. Nothing *could* go wrong. Surely we didn't deserve any more bad luck? This baby had chosen the most unlikely of times to make its entrance into our world, but that had to be for a reason.

We spent a bit more time with Tracy and Chris, but I was itching to get away because I needed something desperately. It was only when we got in the car that I realized all the local shops were shut and my first craving had appeared – I wanted a copy of *Mother & Baby* magazine right away.

Chapter Twenty-three

Chemo countdown

26–27 April 2005

Two days after I found out I was pregnant, Paul was due to start his chemotherapy. We spent the day before buying food that would be easy for him to eat and easy for me to take into hospital to try and stimulate his appetite.

I made a chart to stick on the fridge so that Paul would see where he was with the treatment and how long he had to go. He liked things to be organized in that way, and he liked me to do it for him.

At the top of the sheet, I wrote 'Countdown' then 'Days Remaining'. I wrote down the dates and also how many days of chemotherapy were left. I put in what the tumour marker levels were after each test and any appointments we had at the hospital. Paul had to plan for the first 20-day cycle starting on Tuesday 26 April. His markers at that point were just under 24,000. We called the hospital to confirm that there was a bed available and the nurse said we should get there as soon as possible.

We were met by Dawn, the same nurse we'd had last time.

She was lovely to us and said that she'd saved Paul a side room so that he would be on his own. He had blood tests taken and waited an hour until the doctors arrived. They told him that the scan and injections that needed to be done first were booked for the next day. If the date couldn't be changed to today, then the chemotherapy couldn't start.

Paul was gutted. 'I've psyched myself up for this,' he told them. 'I don't think I can take any delays. I just want this cancer blasted to kingdom come.' He was getting quite upset and I felt guilty because I had other things on my mind as well. I couldn't help with injections or scans or chemo treatment, but I could surely find a nurse in this hospital who would do me another pregnancy test. It would be so wonderful, in the middle of all this awfulness, if we might have a shot at some luck. I wanted Paul to have something to hold onto.

I found a nurse and explained to her that I needed to have the pregnancy test confirmed one way or the other. In the chemotherapy pack we'd been given, it had said that pregnant women shouldn't be in contact with patients during certain types of radioactive treatment so it was important that I found out for sure. The nurse was really nice about it and did two tests for me. Miraculously, in the middle of all this worry, something went right – they were both positive. I'd done four now and they all had the same results. Maybe I could let myself start to believe it soon?

I went back to Paul and found out that he hadn't been so fortunate. The scan and injection would have to be done the next day – and the chemo couldn't start until after that. Paul was devastated – I couldn't imagine how it must feel to steel yourself to face all of that and then be told that it's not going to happen yet. The nurse who did the tests on me pulled me to one side and explained that the injection Paul was due to have when he came back was radioactive. I wouldn't be able to go near him for nine hours, then I'd have to keep a distance of a metre between us for the next two or three days. What a nightmare! It was as if he was in quarantine. How were we going to manage? How could I avoid telling people I was pregnant if they visited Paul and noticed I wasn't going anywhere near him? How could I comfort him if I wasn't allowed to touch him?

Paul said not to worry – the baby was the most important thing. I asked him whether this wouldn't make him feel down. He shook his head. 'Anyway, Linz,' he added, 'I'll be the only bloke walking round the chemo wards with a smile on his face. I've got something I could only have dreamed of a few days ago. I'm going to fight for this baby and I'm going to be there, fit as a fiddle, when it's born.'

We went home exhausted and slept for the rest of the afternoon before starting the whole process again the next morning. On the journey to St James', we sat in silence or went robotically through pointless conversation. Paul was to have an Octreotide Isotope scan. If it was positive (if his tumour 'took it up') then he could get radio-labelled Octreotide therapy, which was something else to add to the armoury. This was the radioactive injection so, bizarrely, I found myself leaving hospital at the very time when I felt I should be with him most.

I came back that night with a jacket potato for Paul – I knew he wouldn't like hospital food, and I needed to feel as though I was doing something for him. There were lots of visitors there, including his friend Pid and his family. Paul had supported Pid when he had battled cancer a few years earlier. I remembered Paul and I talking then about how awful cancer was and how lucky we were; we had sympathized with the way families must feel if they have no stable future in front of them and how everything revolves around uncertainty. Now, it was us in that position. Pid fought successfully – but he had Hodgkin's disease and had been given a revolutionary new treatment with stem cells that had helped him to pull through.

In the midst of all the visitors Paul sat with his cold cap on; it was like a strange kind of high-tech crash helmet. He looked so vulnerable, and I wanted to hold him so much. He said that the first hour wearing it was horrible, that he felt his head was going to explode, but after that his scalp went numb so it wasn't too bad.

It hit me.

This was real.

This was actually happening.

That was my Paul sitting up in bed with a drip attached to his vein sending chemo into his body. He'd be on that drip 24 hours a day for the next three days. It wouldn't stop and we knew it would make him ill; we knew it would take him to the brink before hopefully bringing him back. Would he come back? Would he fall over the edge? I needed to push these thoughts from my mind. I needed to avoid being negative so I told myself that it would work, of course it would work.

It was horrible having to leave Paul; they were very flexible about visiting times, so it was 10.30pm before I finally went. The ward was so peaceful. I got home and tried to think about the baby, about the life I was growing instead of the life that was in danger. Paul's chemo stopped about half an hour after midnight so that he could get his system flushed out and he'd said that he would go outside for a little walk then and give me a call. I stayed up, waiting, and sure enough, about 12.45am, he rang. He was sitting outside the hospital, on a bench in the dark, having a cigarette. I thought back to when I watched someone else standing with their drip, smoking, and how much I hated it. Now the shoe's on the other foot, I supposed he needed his little luxuries. The doctors had told us that Paul's cancer had nothing to do with smoking, and that for him to stop at that point would be so stressful that it could be counter-productive.

I went to bed alone, but couldn't sleep. I needed to focus my mind on something else so I decided to buy another pregnancy test in the morning. They were almost like good luck charms to me, and I had a little collection. Please God, I thought, let this one be positive too and I'll take it as a sign that everything is going to work out fine.

Chapter Twenty-four

'Little Paul'

April–May 2005

It was still positive! I went straight to hospital after I'd done the pregnancy test – my sixth. Paul was in quite good spirits that day, but it was starting to get to other people. His cousin Nicky had been on the phone in floods of tears worried that 'little' Paul looked all helpless. She said that she couldn't stop thinking of him when he was a little kid and she'd looked after him; she wanted to be able to do something now; she wished she could fix it for him. As I comforted her, I was dying to tell her the news that we were having a baby, but I'd decided to wait until I was three months gone in case it went wrong. I didn't want to be responsible for giving people any more sorrow at this time.

Dawn, the nurse, was there helping Paul to put his cold cap on. We got chatting and it turned out in an odd coincidence that we had worked in a salon together about 11 years before. After his visitors had gone, Paul fell asleep. I just sat there looking at him – my gorgeous boy. He was still so beautiful, and I could see past the drips and needles and hospital surroundings. They were just a phase, there to get my Paul better. This time next year, he'd be well and we'd all be together as a family with our baby. There was no denying it was going to be a hell of a fight, but it would be worth it – we could do this.

After about an hour, Paul started to move around and by the time he finally came to, he was in a state. Maybe he was disorientated or had woken up too soon, but he was thrashing about. He dived out of his bed, had a wee in a cardboard cup, and then went all floppy and silent. He sat on the edge of the bed, deep in thought and I could tell he was in a bad way. All of a sudden, the Ronseal advert ('It does exactly what it says on the tin') came on the telly. Paul always used to laugh at it and suddenly he started giggling and the bad mood passed. I loved that about Paul – he could flip from cross to happy in a second. He was so brave, and I loved him so much. I left about 11pm, and got a call from the smoking bench at 12.45am again. That would turn into our ritual whenever Paul had chemo.

The next day was a positive one, I thought, because Paul was due to come home; his first three-day cycle would be over. I got a shock when I went in to collect him. His face was so bloated it looked as though it had been blown up with a pump. He was desperate to get home, but his legs felt dead and heavy with all the fluid that was collected in them. It turned out that he'd put on a stone and a half in three days with all the liquid that had been dripped into him. He was a star with the cold cap that day – while another patient on the ward only managed to put up with the discomfort for 10 minutes, Paul could do between four and five hours a day. I guess that showed how much he loved his hair. I was glad that there was an achievement like that, where he could see he was doing well.

Now came a nerve-racking bit as we were prepared for what to do at home; it was frightening to think there wouldn't be any nurses around, but I'd have to cope on my own. I wrote down the names of all his medication – Allupurinol, Magnesium Glycerophospate, Metaclopromide, Dexamethasone. Not so long ago I didn't even know these things existed, but soon the names would trip off my tongue. It was another language, another world. Paul took the cold cap off 45 minutes early because he just wanted to get home. When we did, I could sense the relief in him. He'd always liked his home comforts, and this environment would hopefully help his recovery. I went to the chart on the fridge and highlighted another day of treatment that had passed. The next important date was Day 8 for his Bleomycin.

The first night at home wasn't as straightforward as I'd hoped. I thought he would just sleep, but he was up all night feeling sick and I couldn't drop off because I was so worried. He got up at 8am, as it was time for his medication, and immediately felt better. It went on like that for a couple of days until he felt not better, but even worse.

'I feel like shit, Lindsey,' he told me. 'I'm on the verge of being sick all the time but nothing's happening. I want to either be sick or not feel sick – it's crap being stuck halfway between. And my fingers – I'm losing sensation in my fingertips.' This was one of the side effects he'd dreaded most because it was the one that could affect his snooker playing. God bless him, he thought he'd be back on the baize any day.

He got up really early every morning and just lay on the sofa for most of the day. On Bank Holiday Monday he was glued to the telly watching Matthew Stevens in the 2005 World Snooker Final; they'd always been close, from the days when they entered all those early tournaments together and Alan and Matt's dad would rent places for them to stay. We had planned to go and support him, but there was no way Paul was well enough to even make the trip, much less cope with all the attention. It would completely drain him and he couldn't afford to waste any energy. In the event Matt lost 18–16.

Paul talked to me about the chemo he'd just been through. 'If only someone could tell you that those three days had some effect,' he said. 'If you knew that the cancer had taken a battering then you could feel positive. It would make it worthwhile. But I can't take any more bad news, Linz. I'd take a downward spiral, I know I would. I hate having to accept this "wait and see" business.'

He'd have to though – we weren't due back at Jimmy's until Wednesday 4 May.

I kept trying to pull Paul back, because he was in danger of disappearing inside himself he was feeling so bad. I kept talking about the baby and telling him everything was going to work out just fine. We got through the next few days and went back to the hospital for the first Bleomycin treatment. Looking back at Paul's hospital notes, I see that they have written: '*Paul has tolerated his first few days of chemotherapy very well. Apart from slight problems sleeping at home and some very mild nausea which settled with his Metaclopramide, he has continued it very well.*' I'm glad they thought so. Maybe Paul understated what it had been like when he was asked, but 'very well' was not how it had felt at all.

He also got the results of his scan back that day, which showed that there was no point in adding radio-labelled octreotide into the mix; the doctors decided just to go ahead with their initial treatment. Paul wasn't too sure how he felt about that. On the one hand, he'd hoped for a wonder drug, but on the other he didn't want to feel any worse by taking something that was unnecessary. It just felt like a maze. There were so many choices, and most of them were taken out of our hands. We didn't know how far we'd gone forwards or whether we were actually going backwards. It was a topsy-turvy world in those clinics and Paul usually expected me to make sense of it all for him.

Then there were the things we hadn't accounted for – things that would have been pretty insignificant for someone who was well, but that could set a cancer patient back almost instantly. That was what faced us when Paul woke up clutching his face in agony one morning. 'Paul!' I cried. 'What is it? What's the matter?' He couldn't speak until the wave of pain had passed a bit.

'It's my mouth and throat, Linz, I've got shooting pains and feel like I'm on fire.' It was a wisdom tooth coming through and setting his throat off – we had to pray it wouldn't turn into tonsillitis. I took his temperature and it was 37.7 degrees, and I was terrified that he had an infection. On top of the chemotherapy, that would be awful – but at least he had an outpatient appointment that day to which his dad was taking him. When he came back, Paul said that he had just been told to keep an eye on things. Knowing how much he hated the idea of hospital admission, I wondered if he had told them the truth about how bad it really was.

We settled down to watch the telly that night – I remember the *Soap Awards* were on and Paul adored his soap operas – and we had fish and chips for tea. He wasn't his usual self; he was all shivery and quiet. At one point he got up and took his own temperature. 'Linz,' he said softly, coming back through, 'It's gone up. It's 38 degrees.' I knew he wouldn't want to hear it but I told him that we had to ring the emergency helpline. 'I'm not going in! I'm not staying in there!' he protested, but he'd have to do as he was told. And the doctor told him what he didn't want to hear – to get in there now.

I drove across town as fast as any ambulance and Paul was told that he'd have to stay in hospital for between two and seven days so that he could be put on an antibiotic drip. He seemed really pissed off, and I did wonder if he sometimes lost sight of the magnitude of all this. Did he know what he was fighting? Did he know that the slightest little thing could knock him back – permanently? I did get a bit frustrated. 'It's not about wanting to stay in your own bed, Paul,' I wanted to shout. 'It's about surviving.'

I went home again to get clothes and toiletries for him and when I got back to the hospital he still wasn't on the drip. I always expected things to happen straight away and was frustrated that I couldn't do more. I stayed another three hours or so feeling relieved that at least he was somewhere there would be an immediate response if anything happened.

I popped in to see him the next morning and he was looking much better but the doctors were still saying he'd have to stay in for a minimum of 48 hours.

I'd just got back home from that visit when there was a call from Paul, his voice cracking. 'Can you come in, Linz?'

Oh God, had something happened? 'Straight away?' I asked, trying to keep calm.

'Yeah. And bring the clippers, babes – my hair's coming out in clumps.'

Chapter Twenty-five

For better, for worse

May–June 2005

I t was just another bit of evidence. Confirmation. When someone you love gets cancer, there's a bit of you thinks it'll be different to anyone else's experience. Chemotherapy will be a walk in the park. They won't be sick. They won't lose their hair.

You always come across someone who thinks they're a cancer expert; someone had told me that you should hope for lots of awful side effects because that means the chemo is working properly. I didn't know what to think. Should I have been glad that Paul's hair was falling out? Did that mean things were going well? You're told at the clinic not to pay much attention to other people's stories because what does or doesn't happen to them might be completely irrelevant for your case. But it was hard not to hope for stories of miracles – I wanted to hear about someone who'd had exactly the same cancer as Paul, got exactly the same treatment, and had been fighting fit for years.

Paul was actually quite chipper about his hair coming out

by the time I got there – mostly because he'd had some good news. Not only was he able to come home because the intravenous antibiotics had done their job, but his tumour markers – which had started off at nearly 24,000 – were down to 13,000. Dr Chester told Paul that he would have been happy with those figures after the second cycle of chemo, never mind the first. This was just the sort of news he needed to get. I went back home and wrote the number up on my little sheet, with 'THINK POSITIVE' scrawled beside it in capitals. When Paul got back, he tried, bless him, he really tried. The news about the markers coming down gave us a real boost. It was something concrete to hold onto, something that couldn't be misinterpreted or confused.

By the time we went back to the oncology clinic on 18 May, Paul blended in with all the other cancer patients – still a bit bloated, hardly any hair, and too much knowledge of the place. We met another bloke called Neil who had also been dealing with an infection. His was an abscess and so bad that he hadn't even been able to get home between chemo cycles, so Paul felt luckier after hearing that.

I soon found out that you can never guess accurately what the patient's mood will be. There were times when if I tried to be 'up', Paul would take it as a slight, an indication that I wasn't bothered enough. Other days, if I seemed quiet he'd complain that if *I* couldn't be positive, what chance did *he* have?

We quite often got good news but the euphoria never lasted very long. I thought that because the markers were down, and because Paul didn't have to put up with the awfulness of the cold cap any more (there was no point once his hair started coming out anyway), that he would be fine. But he wasn't eating much and he was incredibly fed up. Then on the Thursday he went a bit crazy. He started crying out in anxiety, trying to tear the drip from his arm.

'I can't feel free until I get beyond the doors of this hospital,' he screamed at me. 'I'm stuck in here. It's a prison, and everything I have to go through is torture.' He wasn't complaining, he was just trying to make sense of how he felt.

I had thought that the three-day cycles would be relatively easy but I was wrong. We were both exhausted. 'Paul,' I said, 'you've never mentioned what day it is today.'

That made him give a little smile. 'I know what day it is, Linz – how could I not?' Sitting there, we were silent for a while, both of us reflecting on where we were at that time last year. In Jamaica. Making our vows to be husband and wife.

For better or for worse.

Till death us do part.

What a first anniversary. What a way for those vows to take on such significance. I put Paul's hand on my tummy, ignoring the drip that was pumping drugs through him. 'We've plenty more ahead of us, babes,' I reassured him. 'This time next year we won't be celebrating on our own either; we'll have this little one to keep us company. We'll have a five-month-old baby by then, Paul. It'll be beside us and you'll be fit as a fiddle.'

'A baby? It?' he said. 'I'm telling you now, Linz, it's a girl: 6lbs 5oz and the dead spit of me.'

I stayed there a while as we hugged and the mood changed. This tiny little baby inside me was already working some magic; being pregnant put lots of things in perspective. Paul wasn't fighting just for himself – he was fighting for the family we could become.

He was allowed home the next evening and seemed in fairly good spirits. He was beginning to take the initiative and make some decisions on his own. He opted not to take the steroids that were meant to help with the sickness because they seemed to stop him from sleeping. It was the right decision because it turned out that he only had one episode of sickness anyway and did sleep a bit better.

There was more good news from the hospital – four weeks after the start of chemotherapy, his tumour markers were down to 2,760, still incredibly high but miles better than when he started. I could only summarize it by putting 'YIPPEE!' on the chart.

The newspapers and telly were full of one story – Kylie Minogue had been diagnosed with breast cancer. I wrote 'Poor Kylie' in my diary, and Paul remarked how funny it was that he should be watching a story about someone else in the public eye going through the same thing. There were lots of stories about survival rates and remission and what she could expect during chemotherapy. I thought it was useful in helping Paul to understand the process a bit better. He was having it explained to him in relation to someone else, so he could get a bit of distance while he could also relate to it.

He said he felt as though cancer was mentioned everywhere you looked. He talked again about how when anti-smoking ads used to come on telly, he'd often say, 'That'll be me; I'll be the one in three.' You can't take any pleasure in being right about things like that so I teased him again about the fact that he's not psychic; I bet him he was going to be wrong about the sex of the baby.

On 25 May he went back to the oncology unit for a half boost with the Bleomycin. In the following days, his hands were agony, with the joints all swollen from the chemo. He wasn't able to use his fingertips, or flush the loo, or open a bottle of pop, or even open the flip top on the ketchup bottle. But there was no choice – he just had to get through it.

In the clinic there was a poster on the wall quoting the 'one in three' statistic. 'Christ, Lindsey,' Paul said, pointing to it. 'There's a hell of a lot of one in threes in here.' We felt guilty laughing, but it's a lot better than crying.

Paul continued to have trouble with his gums and during his second boost of chemo, he had to be given extra painkillers. I was just praying that we could get through this cycle without infection, but we were actually given more of a boost than that when the news came in that his markers were down to 590. I wrote on the chart: 'FAB!! YOU STRONG BOY!!' It was amazing to look at – everything on that sheet of paper showed that things were going well; of course Paul had been suffering from side effects and it had hardly been plain sailing, but the numbers were coming down and that made everything worthwhile.

Paul's friend Darren Clarke arrived on the day of his next

CT scan (a kind of section by section X-ray that shows up internal tumours) and he was to prove an absolute godsend. They'd been friends since Paul was 10 and during that first bout of chemo, he moved in with us for about three months. He kept Paul occupied – playing pool or darts or watching *Big Brother* – and that gave me some time to get on with my work. It had been hard juggling the salon, college, Paul, the house, hospital, and being pregnant at the same time. People were already asking me how I coped, but I didn't have a magic solution. There honestly wasn't any choice. How could I not cope? What would happen? I didn't have time to sit in a corner crying – I had a baby on the way and Paul to look after, as well as a career and a house to run.

What would have happened if I had decided to just sit around being miserable all the time? If it would have solved something, I'd have given it a try. But I believed that feeling sorry for myself would be a slap in the face for Paul, given all he was coping with. I'd always been brought up to look at problems with a view to solving them: if there was something you could do to make things better, do it; if you couldn't do anything, then there was no point in getting yourself worked up. My mum and dad and Tracy and Chris were an amazing source of support to Paul and me through everything, and I'm sure I wouldn't have coped half as well without them.

Darren Clarke, aka Daz, helped so much over the months. They even played golf when Paul was up to it – when his hands could hold a club. He was still looking towards a future with snooker in it and he worried a lot about the prospect of his hands not improving. I think when Daz was there, I looked at Paul more objectively. I could stand back and watch the way he was describing the treatments to someone else, and I was blown away by his courage.

Everyone you ask says the same. Paul never complained about his illness. He didn't expect special treatment. He carried on living his life as much as he could, playing sport, chatting to his mates, and he didn't obsess about things. Cancer had made him grow up. He was an inspiration. I had pretty much always treated him as my little baby and mothered him – but now I could see just what he was capable of. He always had the ability to amaze me with his mental strength during snooker games, but now he was applying that to real life as well and I was blown away.

As I watched him, I could sense what a great dad he was going to be. When he was able to, he tried to look after me a bit, although he was limited in what he could do without the use of his hands. I think during his illness I realized more than any other time just how well we complemented each other. I didn't give him sympathy in a sloppy way and he didn't moan. If Paul had had someone round him always saying, 'Oh God, this is terrible. Oh God, why did this happen to us?' he would have sunk lower. I had to keep strong, because it kept him strong too.

By the time the next cycle of chemo was due to start on 8 June, we were both really feeling the benefit of Daz being there, and he offered to spend the day with Paul in hospital. Perhaps he was Paul's new good luck charm because what the hospital said that day in his notes was incredible:

*Paul is tolerating his chemotherapy very well. His tumour
markers have fallen down to 590 in the last week. His CT
scan shows almost complete resolution of the previously
identifiable sites of disease in the peritoneum with a few non-
measurable traces remaining, indicating a very good partial
response after just 2 cycles of treatment. I explained this to
Paul today who is obviously delighted. I have told him that
this is certainly as good as and probably much better than any
of us would have anticipated. It does raise the possibility that
this may after all be a germ cell tumour because few other
tumours would respond to this kind of degree to
chemotherapy.*

Paul *was* delighted – this was just what we needed. Not only
was it going well; it was going better than they could ever
have hoped. Also, if the tumour was a germ cell one then the
chances of recovery were pretty good. This was fantastic
news. The only cloud on the horizon was the pain in his
hands. From time to time, he would try to shape his hands as
though holding a snooker cue but they just couldn't do it,
which was heartbreaking. When he mentioned it to the consultant, he was told that he could have the next cycle of
chemotherapy over five days instead of three, which would
reduce the level of pain. Paul didn't even consider it for a second, which shows how horrendous those days must have
been if he preferred to be in agony with his hands.

He slept a lot during those three-day cycles, which meant
there weren't so many visitors; when they did come in, he
was often conked out. Paul preferred less fuss anyway – he

preferred to get the three days over and done with without too many people seeing him, although he was always happy to have Daz around.

By this stage Paul needed a sick bowl next to his bed in hospital and beside him at home wherever he was. He'd really started vomiting a lot. I wrote in my diary: *Poor little man. He doesn't eat much so it's that horrible, gripping process with no sick coming out and you feel like you're choking and not getting any air in your lungs.* He was released from hospital on the Friday evening, with his usual post-chemo look: bloated and with gerbil cheeks. By the early hours of the morning, the nausea had started again in earnest. *Paul's been spitting saliva into a towel for the last hour,* I wrote. *Then it comes ... the gripping, thrusting movement. It's so violent. He's red-faced and there's no oxygen getting in.* I put a cold flannel on the back of his neck and just sat with him until it passed. He always seemed so much better when he finally got the sick up, and an hour later we were walking round the house, having a cup of tea and watching the news. This was the pattern for the next few days.

The doctors said that they were amazed that the tumour had shrunk so quickly and at how well Paul tolerated chemo, then in the next breath they said they might give him more. I said to Paul: 'Get it while the going's good. While you feel like shit, you may as well feel like shit for a while longer knowing that it's actually making you well.'

He usually took these sorts of little speeches from me really well, but this time he turned and hissed, 'It's easy to say, Lindsey, when it's not happening to you.'

I squeezed his hand, but I wanted to scream: 'No, Paul! It isn't easy for me. I'd take this from you if I could, I'd take it all, because you're my world. I'm keeping strong because we can't afford to fall apart. We can't let this thing in or it will take over, and where will we be? Where will our baby be if this has eaten us both up?' Perhaps me being positive all the time was grating on him – I'd worried about it before, and no doubt I'd worry about it again.

There was more good news though – Paul's tumour markers were down to 237, about a tenth of what they had been to start with. 'MIND OVER MATTER!' I wrote on the chart. Daz stayed around until August before he had to get back home to Leicester to see his son, and he definitely helped to keep Paul sane through that whole period.

Meanwhile, on Saturday 18 June, I was exactly 12 weeks pregnant. Nothing was stopping this baby – it was solid, and it kept on growing. Now I was past the miscarriage stage I could tell close family and friends about it. I went to Blackpool for a night out with some friends and Paul had the boys over. All our mates were over the moon and speculating on who the baby would look like, which characteristics it would get from both of us, and teasing Paul about changing nappies and so forth. Seeing his friends made him feel more normal again. I stopped writing my diary at that point, because it felt as though things were on the up. I was proud of us – we were getting through and we were winning.

Chapter Twenty-six

Our baby

From the minute I found out that I was having a baby, Paul was so excited. It was like all his Christmases had come early. I think he thought he'd done all his hard work, so he could just bask in the glory of being a daddy-in-waiting. He had that cock-of-the-walk look about him – I could see what he was thinking: ' I've made her pregnant! My sperm works!'

When we could, when Paul was well enough, we loved to do normal baby-related things so that we weren't Paul the cancer patient and Lindsey his poor wife any more – we were Paul and Lindsey expecting their first baby.

Early on, we bought a book each. I got one on pregnancy and what to expect, while Paul bought one on babies' names. The baby was due on New Year's Eve and Paul said, 'If it's a girl shall we have Evie as a name?' We liked Holly and Jessica too, and I loved Harrison for a boy, so that was our short list.

We bought all the magazines on pregnancy and your baby and what to expect, and at night we lay in bed reading what was happening to the baby that week and what would be happening the week after. I'd lie there telling him, 'It's got fingers now!' We were absolutely amazed by it all.

Even though my sister Tracy had children and so had lots of other friends and family, it's amazing how different it is when it's you. It just seems so incredible that this tiny little thing that starts from nothing is growing inside you every second.

As the weeks went by, I was desperate to have a bump – I think that's always the case with your first. You just want to show the world, let everybody know that you've managed it. However, I didn't even look pregnant until I was about 18 or 19 weeks. Because of Paul's illness, the pregnancy took a back seat a lot of the time. I don't even have many pictures of me over the nine months I carried the baby because I was always the one holding the camera. There was a voice in the back of my mind saying: take photographs of Paul, take lots of photographs of Paul – maybe it was my pessimistic side.

We had quite a few antenatal classes – some of them together and some just for mums-to-be. Paul got into a bit of a flap before the first one. He said, 'Oh God, what are they going to do? What are they going to expect me to do? Will I look daft? Will they all know stuff that I don't?' I had to remind him that I was clueless about it all too.

I remember that class as though it was yesterday. Paul had no hair at this stage, so he was wearing a lovely, soft, woolly hat to keep his head warm. 'What's it going to be like, Linz? Is it all going to be young girls? Will I be the only bloke there?' he kept asking me.

He needn't have worried; everyone was so friendly. The

nurse who took the class put us at our ease straight away. Two women in the class were further on than me, one was at the same stage, and one five weeks behind. They ranged from 18 to their 30s. We all had to introduce ourselves and when it got to us, Paul plucked up the courage to talk. He never presumed that anyone knew who he was. He said, 'Hi, I'm Paul. I've actually got cancer and Lindsey has been absolutely fantastic through it all. I should be looking after her; it's the one time in her life she should be spoiled, but when I get better I'm going to repay her and do everything for her.' I told him to shut up, but what he had said was just lovely.

We then had to pair up with another couple and do a quiz to find out about each other. We got talking to one couple in particular; the woman was five weeks behind me. What was nice was that we were all there for something so good and positive that Paul and I were able to forget for a little while what else we had to deal with.

It was nice just to have a laugh as well. At one point, the nurse got a pair of big trackie bottoms out of a cupboard and said, 'I need a lad to help me here.' One of them went up and she helped him to put them on. Then she said, 'This is what your partner will go through for the next six months or however long they've got.' She started throwing bags of sugar and tins inside the tracksuit trousers, saying, 'This is the placenta, and this is how much the baby weighs, and this is what the baby's weight will go up to.' This particular lad had been saying earlier, 'How hard can it be? How hard can having a baby be?' Now he was holding the bottoms and the nurse said, 'You know what? This is what your wives and partners are carrying around, and you're only having to deal with the weight issue, you haven't got the hormones and everything else inside those trousers!'

She was really funny. Then she started taking things out of the trousers and said, 'You're giving birth now! There goes your water breaking, there goes the baby, there goes the placenta!' But she left some of it in the trackies just to show the men that it doesn't all go straight away – I think she terrified a few of the women too.

Paul sat there calmly watching it all, laughing with the rest of us. He always said he wasn't very confident in social situations but now and again he would come out with something that showed his great sense of humour. While the lad was standing there, still with tins and sugar down his trousers, Paul said, 'All right, fair enough. Now tell us what we really want to know – when does your wife get back down to a size 8?'

Everyone burst out laughing and I exclaimed, 'Paul! I can't believe you just said that!' He said all the other lads were probably wondering the same thing.

We laughed a lot that night and when we came home we agreed it wasn't so bad; there hadn't been anything to get nervous about at all. We enjoyed making new friends there and being sociable.

When we went back the following week it was all about pain relief. The nurse asked, 'Does anyone know any massage?' I shouldn't have admitted it, but I put my hand up and said that, actually, I taught it. I ended up taking the whole class! All these men were getting taught by me how to massage their wives' backs and I didn't even get one myself!

At the next class we had a tour round the hospital facilities at Dewsbury. I wasn't actually going to give birth there but all the other women in the class were, so we just tagged along. I had chosen to go to Leeds to have the baby because Paul was having his treatment there and I thought that if he was poorly when I went into labour, at least we'd be in the same building. Hopefully he'd be able to get to the birth, even if someone from the oncology unit had to help him.

Walking round Dewsbury, I thought it had a lovely atmosphere. There were lots of different options depending on how you wanted to have your baby. I especially liked the room with the birthing pool. Paul asked if blokes were allowed to get in the pool as well and the midwife said that was fine. You could have the baby in there, or relax in the water to relieve the pain then get out when it was time.

Next the midwife brought out the gas and air. I wasn't so sure about that, but Paul was up for having a go. I said, 'Are you sure you're going to be all right, babes? You're taking so much else, this could just push you over.' He wouldn't listen, though, and he started sucking on the tube thing and everyone was watching and waiting to see what would happen. In the first few minutes, Paul said there was nothing, he didn't feel any different. Then it hit him and he started laughing, saying he could feel it and it was really nice! I had a go and he was right, so I decided that I would probably have a bit of that when the time came. The midwife said I should pop it in my birth plan – but I didn't have a birth plan! I still didn't really feel pregnant, to tell the truth. All the other girls had little notebooks and folders and they had all decided what they wanted it to be like, what method of delivery they wanted, what pain relief, what music they wanted to be play-ing. All I could think was that if I needed something on the day, I'd have it; if I didn't, I wouldn't.

After I thought about it a bit more, I decided that I wanted to stay moving around for as long as possible and not lie down on a hospital bed. I suppose my final decision was made when we got to the delivery suite – all sterile and clinical and sparkling. The others all looked horrified but I said, 'Oh, *that's* what I want – a nice clean place where I won't catch anything!'

The following week we went on a tour around St James' maternity wards. Maybe it's changed since then but at that time, even though it was a teaching hospital, there weren't any options. There were just delivery rooms – no birthing pool or anything – so it turned out I had no choice after all. I knew I wanted to stay at home for as long as possible, then move around when I got to the delivery room, maybe taking a fitness ball with me. The only other thing I knew was that I wanted Paul to cut the cord. Bless him – he said he'd have a go even though he was squeamish. His only other comment was that he wanted to 'stay up the top end and not go down there'. He just 'didn't fancy it'!

I decided I didn't want to breastfeed – well, I should say, Paul preferred me not to breastfeed. He kept joking 'boobs aren't for babies, they're for men' and as I wasn't too worried either way, that was that. Another reason for bottlefeeding was so that Paul could feed the baby too. I really wanted him to have that special time from the start. I suppose I wanted life to be as normal as possible, and that included my husband bonding with our baby in every way, so I agreed that, unless I felt really different after I gave birth, I'd bottlefeed.

That meant all my decisions were made. However, there was a voice in the back of my mind that worried that I was going to follow in my sister Tracy's footsteps – she had had to have an emergency Caesarean. I really didn't want a section but it was as well to prepare myself for the worst. It didn't matter – there was no way I could have predicted what was going to happen anyway.

Chapter Twenty-seven

What's the sex?

I didn't have my first scan till I was 15 weeks pregnant. Generally they do one at 12 weeks, but because I was transferring to another hospital for the delivery my notes had to be sent over and that caused the delay. I asked Paul to come along with me on the day and he agreed, although it meant going back to St James' on a non-chemo day.

There was a bit of waiting about because I had to get some blood tests done as well. Some people stared at Paul because he was bald and it was obvious that he had cancer. It's not just about the hair loss I guess – there's a look to cancer patients. You know they're going through the mill. I wasn't sure whether the people in that waiting room recognized Paul – maybe they'd read he had cancer, maybe they'd seen us in the papers talking about how happy we were that I was pregnant. Or maybe they had loved someone who had been through the same. You don't know other people's stories, but sometimes you get a glimmer of what might be there.

As well as pregnant women and their partners, there were

parents there with little babies waiting to see a doctor. I looked at some and thought: 'Poor you.' They looked at us and thought the same, I guess. Were they thinking how awful it must be to be fighting cancer when you've got a baby on the way? Were they wondering how we were going to cope? Or were they just thinking, 'Oooh, look, it's Paul Hunter off the telly'?

I kept asking Paul if he was all right because he had been quite sick earlier that day. He said he was but usually we carried a bucket or a bag for him to vomit into and we hadn't brought one that day because he didn't want to sit in a public place with it on his knee. I know he felt quite vulnerable without it. Paul had also been warned he was anaemic and there was a chance he could pass out, but fortunately he survived that waiting room without either passing out or being sick.

At an earlier appointment, when the midwife had been testing my blood pressure and checking for the baby's heartbeat, she had scared the life out of me by saying: 'Oh. I can't find the heartbeat today.' I almost collapsed at those words. There was so much pressure on. I was thinking, 'This baby has just got to be all right. It's just got to be.' I had to make a perfect baby. Paul almost looked more upset and worried about that than he did about his own problems. I was still thinking, please let it be OK, please let it be OK, when the midwife announced that it was fine after all and sometimes it all depended on where the baby was lying.

Another of my worries was that maybe I was having a phantom pregnancy. Perhaps because we'd wanted it so much, and because I knew it would make everyone feel better, I'd just imagined myself pregnant? I didn't feel pregnant. You couldn't see a bump. I'd been a tiny bit more tired at teatime around weeks seven and eight, so I'd had a nap for an hour or so, which I never normally do. I'd maybe felt sick one or two mornings but nothing came up. That was the extent of my pregnancy problems. Was there really a baby in there? I wouldn't have been at all surprised if someone had turned round and said: 'Lindsey, it's all in your mind.'

When I was about 13 or 14 weeks pregnant, a client at work was chatting away and mentioned that when she'd gone for her 12-week scan, they told her that the baby had died. I couldn't stop dwelling on that and thinking, please, don't let that have happened. Maybe that was why I didn't have any pregnancy symptoms. This was another reason why I was so desperate to have a scan – to set my own mind at rest and to let Paul see everything was fine (if it was).

They say the images are better the fuller your bladder is, so I'd drunk litres and litres of water and I was absolutely bursting. They started to put the gel on my tummy. I was holding my breath and didn't dare look at first but before I knew it, I could hear them saying, 'There you go – everything's perfect.'

Paul was just stunned. He was staring at the screen and watching the baby. Our baby. Our son, I soon decided, because while we were watching, all of a sudden it put its little thumb up. I said: 'Oh my God! It's definitely a boy, sticking his thumb up at his daddy like that!' We got loads of pictures, including one in a little cardboard frame. Paul loaded one on his mobile as a screensaver and we sent it off straight away to show Paul's parents and my parents and friends.

I was so relieved that there was actually a baby there! There was another decision to make, though. At one of the antenatal classes, the midwife had told us about the different blood tests you could get done at various stages. She talked about the triple test and the way it could flag up your risk of having a baby with Down's syndrome or other handicaps. I thought that seemed like a good idea and decided that I'd have the blood test done. We were told the blood test would come back either 'high' or 'low'; it would give us an idea of the likelihood of problems, then we could make a decision about whether to have an amniocentesis test. I was also told that if I did have the amnio, there was a risk of miscarriage even if the baby was fine. I didn't really know what to do. Paul didn't know much about those sorts of things and he said I should decide.

We went home and over the next few days had to talk about tests. Paul said: 'If the test comes back high, what do we do?' I told him we'd have to consider another test that came with a risk of miscarriage. 'Would you want to get rid of the baby, Paul?' I asked him. 'Because, personally, I wouldn't. If this is the only chance we have to have a baby together, I'm not bothered how it turns out. Obviously I want it to be perfect, but I don't think we should put ourselves through all that and maybe have a miscarriage of a perfectly healthy baby.'

To be honest, if you'd asked me a year before, I'd have said: 'I'm having the triple test and that's that. If it comes back high risk, I'm having an amnio, and if that comes back positive, I'm probably having an abortion.' I couldn't imagine bringing up a disabled baby and I don't think Paul would have wanted to either, but, because of the situation we were in, we thought if that was the only chance of us having our own baby, we would take it.

We asked ourselves what we would do if it came back with a high risk of maybe 1 in 30. What about the 29 times it would be fine? Were we willing to risk losing a healthy baby? Then we decided to stop being so negative. Hadn't we had enough bad luck? There was a much better chance of our baby being healthy than having problems. It would have been a different story if Paul hadn't been poorly but he was, and we had to factor that into things. I can't deny that I always had a tiny niggling worry, but everything seemed to be progressing well so I opted for my positive thinking approach and ignored the little voice in my head.

The next few weeks went by and Paul was due for another three days of chemotherapy. I remember thinking: I hope he's going to be all right to come and see the scan with me at 20 weeks. He actually got out of hospital the day before the appointment.

I didn't want to know whether it was a boy or a girl but Paul didn't agree. He said: 'Let's get one of those 3D scans and see the baby properly.' I didn't want to because they're meant to be so much clearer and we would probably be able to see what sex it was. When we went back for the next scan, all the measurements were fine and everything was going along just as it should.

I said: 'I don't want to know, but can you tell what sex the baby is?' Immediately the doctor said: 'Yes, I can.' I had to go for a wee because I was bursting as usual, and Paul teased me: 'While you're away, I'm going in again to find out whether it's a boy or a girl!' I told him he'd better not, but when I got back, he said, 'I've been in!' I told him he'd better be joking and it turned out he was. I was even more sure that it had to be a boy because of the way the doctor said straight away that he could tell – he must have seen a willy! But Paul said it wasn't, that he was sure it would be a girl, and he was betting on her weighing 6lbs 5oz.

Everything just toddled along after that. I was still working, still dealing with Paul's visits to the hospital, and still not really feeling pregnant. I remember asking the midwife if I could come to appointments every four weeks instead of every two nearer the end because I was so busy, but she said that it was important that I still checked in. I couldn't get out of hospitals and doctors' visits even when I tried.

Chapter Twenty-eight

Normal

June–September 2005

The antenatal classes and all the growing excitement about the baby meant that we had a distraction from cancer treatments. It finally seemed as if things were going our way. Paul's next results were even more reason to celebrate – on 22 June, his tumour markers were down to 114. The doctors said the rate at which they were falling indicated 'an ongoing excellent response to therapy' – which was just what Paul needed to hear. He had a low platelet count at that stage but was feeling pretty good.

It just kept getting better and better – by July, and the beginning of his fourth chemotherapy cycle, the markers were down to 34 and then 18 at the end. This was working. We were getting there, slowly, painfully, but – thank God – successfully. The doctors wanted him to go ahead with a further two cycles of chemo after that to get him down still further. They said that the drop had been 'pretty spectacular' but that there was still room for improvement. Paul was upset – to say the least – at the prospect of more chemo; I had to emphasize that it was because he was doing so brilliantly that the consultants thought he should go ahead with more, as there was a chance things could get even rosier.

The fifth cycle was booked to start on 10 August, and this time it would be without Bleomycin, as Paul had already been given the full permitted dose. To give us both something to look forward to we decided to plan a holiday to Rhodes afterwards. We knew it would be different to any other break we'd had before, but we'd be happy to sit quietly, on our own, relaxing. There were problems getting holiday insurance. Paul was warned about the possibility of picking up infections between bouts of chemo, as the body can't fight things off in the normal way, but Dr Chester supported our case to go on holiday and wrote to the insurance company saying that Paul was having 'an excellent response to his treatment'. We were told to make sure that we knew where the nearest specialist oncology centre was if there did seem to be a problem, or to call Dr Chester directly from Rhodes.

Paul's fourth session of chemo was awful. The doctors could tell him all they liked that he was tolerating it well because he was young, but the reality was that it was horrendous. We still planned to go to Rhodes, but Paul was too ill to attend his sister's wedding in Cyprus on 27 July. That was one of our worst days so far. While Leanne was getting married hundreds of miles away, Paul was sick 30 times in 36 hours. He had severe thrush in his throat from all the vomiting and was the lowest I'd ever seen him.

I could hear him trying to be sick in our bathroom again,

but there was barely even any saliva left. I didn't know whether to go in or not.

Then I heard the sobbing.

Paul had hardly cried through all of this, and I didn't know what to do. Maybe he wanted to be left alone. Maybe he wanted to be comforted. I had to do what my heart told me, and I rushed in.

'Darling, what is it?' I asked, pulling him towards me.

'What the fuck do you think it is, Lindsey?' he said. 'I'm tired. I'm so fucking tired of all this.'

'But you're winning, babes, you're winning,' I told him.

'Does this look like I'm fucking winning?' he asked, with great gulps of tears choking him.

I didn't really want to look.

But I did.

He was a shadow of himself.

He had no hair.

He was grey.

His eyes were sunken.

He had lost weight but was bloated too.

His hands and fingers were numb.

He was freezing but sweating.

One side of his face was swollen and the eye was completely bloodshot from the sickness.

His veins were wrecked from all the injections and blood tests and I could see needle marks all over him.

His lips were cracked, his skin was an unholy colour, and the old, greyish-white bathrobe that seemed to have become his uniform was caked in vomit.

I couldn't help myself – I started crying. 'I must be as bad as I think I am,' Paul said.

We sat there, together, in the bathroom and cried and cried and cried like we'd never cried before. All the fear and relief and panic and hope of the last months came together in one burst of emotion and the only way to get it out was to sit there wailing together.

After we cried it all out, I said to him: 'Paul, we can't do this again. We can't let it get us. We've cried, we need to move on.'

'I know, Linz, I know,' he replied. 'I didn't think I'd ever cry like that anyway – but it's out now, it's over and done with.'

We hugged again and I held his face in my hands as I said, 'You know what, Paul Hunter? You're still absolutely gorgeous!' We sat there together for ages on the bathroom floor, just cuddling. Paul tried to be sick again a few more times, and I felt closer to him than I ever had before.

When we went back to get Paul's tumour marker test results in August, the doctor said they had stayed at 18. 'What does that mean?' I asked. 'It means that there's no point in having a sixth cycle,' Dr Chester said. 'You've turned a corner, Paul. We can only hope that this means things are looking up.' Paul was told that he didn't need to come back until we returned from our holiday but he was to have one last blood test before we left and he'd get the results on his return. When we got home that day, I wrote at the end of my fridge poster: 'WELL DONE!! WE ARE PROUD OF YOU!! FINISH!! ALL CLEAR SUPERMAN!!'

I was 24 weeks pregnant when we flew away to Rhodes

for our last holiday before the baby was born. It was a beautiful time, and in many ways we felt as though the baby was already there – Paul would rub my tummy all the time and talk to it every day. It was like a second honeymoon. He was so happy after being told about his markers that we even started to make love again.

Three nights before we were due to go home, walking back to our hotel, Paul pulled me back. It was a beautiful, warm night. Everything felt perfect. He held me close and we kissed.

'Lindsey?' he said.

'What, babes?' I answered, wanting to hold onto this moment for such a long time.

'I don't think it's gone.'

'What? What do you mean?'

'The cancer. It hasn't gone,' he repeated.

'Of course it has! What about your tests? Don't say things like that, Paul. Stay positive – you've got to stay positive.' I was almost crying by now. I was trying to pull away from him, get back to the hotel, get back to how we had been minutes before, but he wouldn't let me go.

'Lindsey, listen,' he said, with the same weird look in his eye that I had seen the day he was going to tell his mum and dad that he had cancer. 'It's coming back. And next time will make what's gone before seem like a picnic.'

'Oh, Paul,' I wept. 'Don't. Don't.'

'I haven't been all the way to hell yet. But that's where I'm going.'

With that he started to walk away. The magic had been

broken. I tried to talk to him about it that night, the next day, the day after, but he wouldn't say anything else. It was as if he had just made an announcement, that what he had said was fact.

I felt a chill go up my spine.

What I didn't know was that he was right. How could he possibly have known? Was there some sign, some nagging little internal pain that he wasn't telling me about? He never let on.

We went back to Jimmy's a couple of days after getting home. There were the usual delays, the usual time-consuming bothers, but when we went into Dr Chester's office, I was convinced we were going to be told good news. Apart from what Paul had said at the end of our stay, the holiday had been such a breath of fresh air. Now, all we needed was something positive to keep our spirits up.

The three of us went through the usual greeting, and chatted a bit about the holiday, but inside I was screaming – 'Let us know; let us know the numbers!'

'Well, Paul,' said the doctor at last. 'The results from before your holiday aren't quite as good as we would have hoped.'

That was OK, I told myself. We had been told at the beginning of all this that people who were perfectly healthy could have marker figures of up to 30 at times. The last two tests had stayed at 18 – were we up to 25, 30 now?

'This time, they're coming in at …' he looked at the sheet

of paper in Paul's file as if he had never seen it before, 'Over 500. I'm afraid it looks as if there's been a relapse.'

'What happens now?' Paul and I both asked at the same time. I could barely breathe, my chest felt so tight.

There was a pause.

'More chemotherapy.'

I couldn't believe it. Paul was going to have to do it all over again. Just as he'd said – back to hell. We were told that he couldn't have the same type of chemo as his body would now be immune to it. It would have to be a different type. I couldn't take it all in. I just hadn't seen that one coming.

Paul was absolutely devastated. I think he felt that he was a man and he shouldn't cry in front of the doctors, but I also think that he was being defiant. Cancer doctors and nurses seem to think that the person with cancer has to accept it before they can move on and they are constantly asking the patient to say what they think is happening. They want you to explain it, to look ahead to what is in front of you and to be aware of the implications of the diagnosis. Paul and I were quite proud that we usually did our crying in private, but that day when he was told it had come back, he waited until we were right down the hospital corridor and then he wept as if the world was coming to an end.

The following week, a CT scan showed that there was no huge bulk of the disease visible. Dr Chester said that a tiny bit of the cancer must have been left in Paul's body last time – tiny, but enough to grow and enough to send him reeling. And the tumour markers? They were now up to 5,000.

After that, it was as though something in Paul had broken.

He would make little comments, tiny remarks that showed he was thinking it through. Quite often, when I was scared, I would check his lips in the middle of the night to see if they had gone blue, to see if he was still breathing. One night, when I'd thought he was asleep, I was holding my hand over his mouth to see if I could feel the warmth of his breath. Suddenly he grabbed it, opened his eyes and looked at me.

'What are you doing, Lindsey?' he asked. 'I'm checking you're alive, babes,' I said. 'Of course I'm bloody alive!' he snapped, and I was relieved to hear the tone.

He still had a lot of fight left in him; this was the Comeback Kid of the snooker table, and I didn't doubt he'd keep on fighting this opponent with everything he had.

Chapter Twenty-nine

Hard labour

September–December 2005

Instead of coming back from our holiday to a period of remission, Paul had to gather his strength to start yet another cycle of chemo that would be administered every three weeks right into January 2006. Darren came back to stay again, which was a huge help, but every treatment seemed to get harder than the ones that went before. Sometimes Paul couldn't even summon the energy to get dressed when it was time to drive to the hospital. He'd just keep his pyjamas and slippers on and slip a jacket on top.

Wednesday mornings spent in that horrible waiting room were utterly soul-destroying. On every second pale-blue PVC chair sat a bald patient, accompanied by a friend or relative. There were the same magazines on the coffee table that had been there on our first visit back in March. In the corner of the room there was a cupboard with items that cancer patients could buy to help them get through their treatment, but all I remember is the same three pink bandannas that had been there since we first came to the unit. They came to symbolize for me everything that was vile about that place.

We often had a two-hour break after the blood tests were taken and before the chemo could start, so we went to the nearby Thackeray Medical Museum. There are only so many times you can go round a place like that, but they had a café where the ladies were lovely and they got to know Paul. 'Your bacon sarnie's on the way, love,' they'd shout when they saw him, and they never forgot to lay out the brown sauce. Little things like that meant a lot, lightening the load for just a few seconds. I was finding it harder and harder to keep his spirits up, because in private, I was desperately worried myself. Things didn't look good. I wouldn't allow myself to think the worst – I just couldn't go there – but it got harder and harder to find positive things to say as the days went by.

The experience you have as a cancer outpatient takes over the whole of your life. Paul was never good with needles or injections, but he became an expert after a while. Jabs and having bloods done and lines run through him had become run of the mill, but there was still a huge difference between it being done properly or not. It's never a nice experience but sometimes, for Paul, it was a nightmare. If he had an appointment, Paul would often go to the outpatients department first and ask one of the more experienced nurses there to put in the cannula for him rather than risk getting someone else who would stab at his veins for ages without getting the tube in. Paul would slip into the clinic to see who was on duty and sometimes he would frown and say, 'Oh, I'm not having her do it, Linz. She's rubbish. I'll be there for ages and end up having to make her feel better when she keeps getting it in the wrong place!'

One nurse got it really off the mark one day when trying to get an IV in, and she hit a nerve; Paul's fingers went all funny and I knew he was having a hard time controlling himself, it was so sore.

It's funny, because you sometimes feel that because the person you love is dealing with cancer – often terminal – that they should be able to handle anything. They've got the worst already, so anything else should be manageable. You could almost see some of the staff thinking, You've got cancer, you're dying, so why are you whingeing about a needle being stuck in? But the little things still matter, and no one should forget that.

We often wondered why the district nurse couldn't just come to our house and do the blood tests and get them sent off before the clinic appointment, but apparently there are different machines that check the tumour markers and you need to be tested by the same one each time. The only way Paul could sometimes change the routine was to go into Jimmy's on a Tuesday and have his blood tests done that day so that the doctors had them to hand first thing on Wednesday morning.

When we had an appointment to see a doctor, it became the entire focus of the day. You never knew how long anybody else would be – you never knew how long *you* would be. Someone else would go in front of Paul and we'd think, It's us next. It could be five minutes before they came out, or it could be half an hour. That could be the day the patient in front of you was told they had weeks to live, or that they were in remission. In those rooms, lives were being shattered or little glimmers of hope were being offered. Maybe it's selfish but when the person you adore is being kept waiting, you can't think about anyone else. I know that everyone was in the same boat, but this was all we had. I guess it was the same for other patients – I'm sure there were times when Paul went in to see the doctor and others sat there thinking, God, what's taking *him* so long?

If you only go to hospital once in a blue moon these things probably wouldn't bother you; when you go every week, it's another matter. They always said to us in Jimmy's, 'Well, we have a meeting every Wednesday morning and you just have to accept the fact that it can overrun.' I wanted to scream at them, 'So, have it on the Tuesday night!' Those days were so frustrating and so stressful. It didn't matter what we did, we would feel it all bubbling up.

The fact that it was all so inflexible became an issue for us. Paul would go in for a three-day treatment on the Wednesday, Thursday and Friday, which would mean he'd be feeling rotten all weekend too. I once asked if he could have it on a Tuesday, Wednesday and Thursday because then he could recuperate on the Friday and hopefully feel a bit more like himself on the Saturday – which was often when his friends came round as they were off work. They said, no, it had to start on a Wednesday. When I asked why, I was just fixed with a steely glare and told, 'It always is. It just is.'

Having said that, Paul and I recognized that they had a job to do and most of them did it brilliantly; it's just that you focus on your own experience so much that every minute detail is magnified and you go over it time and time again.

Some of them try harder than others – there were certain nurses who always made sure Paul was in a side room on his own, for example. You presume that they are doing all they can and they do have a horrible workload to deal with – but this is your world, this is all you have. This was the tiny little scrap of life that Paul had left, and I wanted it to be perfect, not tied up with other people's meetings and nurses who couldn't put intravenous lines in.

If someone told me now that I had cancer, I don't know what I'd do. I've seen it full on. Is that how you want to spend your final days? I don't think I could go through that if I was to end up as wrecked as Paul became at the end, especially if doctors said that any treatment won't cure it but might give you a couple of extra months: I think I'd say no. I've seen it all at first hand. I'm a fighter but I wouldn't go through all of that for just another couple of months.

It was hard for Paul, there's no denying that, but he wasn't the sort of person who would ever have considered ending it all. Neither was I. People ask me the question – would I have helped him to end it all? Maybe if Paul had been constantly ill, unable to do anything at all, with no good moments at any point … I don't know. If it was what he wanted. I can't really answer because he wasn't that sort of person; he never considered it an option. When you're still here, you always have a little bit of hope even if it's getting smaller all the time.

At the end of each three-day cycle of chemo, Paul seemed to be sicker and sicker. His feet got very cold this time round and he would have to wear big thermal socks to keep them warm. Also, he had no eyelashes left at all, so he often got tiny specks of dust in his eye and I had to help him get them out. Of all the things we take for granted, you never think about eyelashes particularly – until you don't have them.

The snooker season started up again and on 9 October 2005, Paul bravely turned up to play at Preston Guildhall. Although he failed to win a match that day, he had the crowd behind him all the way. During that entire 2005/6 season he didn't miss a match, even when he was turning up at the table with no feeling in his fingertips, with no hair, with stomach pains, wearing his thermal socks, and getting thinner by the day because he was being sick so much and had no appetite. I always said to him that if he felt up to it, he should go for it, and if he had to pull out of a tournament, people would understand – but he never let anyone down. He just got on with it. He never once walked away from the table and left a match unfinished. He was always shattered afterwards but glad that he had given it a go, and his dignity and professionalism throughout that season won him the respect of players and fans worldwide.

Of course, his game suffered – there's no way he was playing with his usual skill and flair, and that meant he lost all but one of his matches during the 2005/6 season and slipped out of the top 32 ranked players in the world. In most sports, if a player experiences an illness for a long period of time his prominence and ranking in his chosen sport is protected by a constitutional law, which allows him to take time out. Not in snooker.

Brandon approached the snooker authorities and asked if it was possible to freeze Paul's ranking for the next season while he finished his cancer treatments so that he didn't slip too far down the scale. All of the players seemed happy for him to do this, but for some reason the powers within the game took an age to make a decision. In hindsight, it was a move they could easily have approached Paul with during the difficult season he had already had to play through. When it did come up for a vote, unbelievably a number of people voted against it. I'd like to know who they were – some people just don't have a charitable bone in their body. Finally, halfway through 2006, they agreed to freeze his ranking but frankly, it was too late for Paul. We had far more important things to worry about by then.

In November 2005, halfway through the cycle, we had the all-important meeting to find out what his tumour markers were. The level had been 5,000 when we got back from Rhodes and it was down – but only to 2,200. Paul stared at the floor, his shoulders hunched, and didn't respond. I had to ask all the questions: 'What does it mean? What do we try next? Surely it's good that it's dropped a bit?' When the doctor said that Paul should continue the chemo through December as planned, I winced. How much could one person take? Physically and mentally, Paul was starting to fall apart before my eyes – but his fighting spirit was still in there somewhere and he agreed to carry on.

*   *   *

I felt guilty because I'd hardly been paying any attention to my pregnancy. I attended the routine appointments and picked up a few bits and pieces of baby clothing and so forth, but apart from that, all my energy was focused on Paul and his treatments. I suppose I was lucky because I was my own boss, to a large extent, with all my different jobs. I still taught at the college every Tuesday and worked in the salon most days, but people would bend over backwards to cover for me on days when I couldn't make it because I had to be with Paul.

When I got to 20 weeks, the expected delivery date was brought forward to 27 December. At this point we still liked the name Evie for a girl and Harrison for a boy (of course, Paul was still insisting it was a girl and I was convinced it was a boy). As the weeks went by, I cut my hours down a little bit at the salon, maybe taking some time off during the day and then going back at night-time, but I was still working when I was 39 weeks pregnant. It didn't feel like a long pregnancy because I didn't show for ages and there were so many other things on my mind.

Paul and I used to love Christmas, but this year it took second place. We kept saying to each other: 'We're getting a baby and that's the biggest present we could ever have.' I was desperately hoping that the baby would be born on time but it was all quite bizarre. I remember everyone saying that you just know when the baby is coming, you just know, but I hadn't been pregnant before so I had no idea what I was supposed to be looking out for. I was in for a few shocks along the way.

I decided not to go into the salon on Christmas Eve as I'd

been working more or less every day up to then. Paul and I had a routine we always followed on 24 December and we didn't see any reason to change it. I got myself dressed and then started loading all the presents I'd bought for everyone into the car. Paul was having a drink, which was fine with me. It was good for him to relax when he felt well enough, and I so wanted him to enjoy this Christmas. Once or twice the thought jumped into my head that it could be his last, but I immediately banished it and made myself think about something else.

I was just walking backwards and forwards carrying all the gifts from the dining room to the car, when all of a sudden there was a gush of liquid between my legs. I seemed to have wet my pants! I shouted, 'Paul! I keep weeing myself. It won't stop, my pants are really wet.' He said: 'No! What's all that about?' and I told him that the baby must be pushing on my bladder, which is what it felt like.

I went upstairs and changed my pants and when I came back down, I said: 'You know, Paul, I'm feeling a bit odd. Every time I bend over to pick up a present, things feel weird.' I truly didn't guess what was happening because I'd got it into my head that first babies are always late – and they'd changed my dates anyway so there was some uncertainty about the exact due date.

I wet myself and had to change my knickers a few more times that morning, but we just got on with things. Even though I'd been to antenatal classes, I didn't dream for a second that it was my waters breaking; I expected that to be something more dramatic. We got in the car and drove round dropping off the presents for everyone. I didn't have any niggly pains or the other symptoms I'd been warned to watch out for, so I was none the wiser when we went to bed on Christmas Eve.

I can't remember exactly what I felt on Christmas morning – just uncomfortable, I suppose. No matter what position I tried, I couldn't get myself comfy. I didn't think it was labour though. The plan for the day was that we'd go to my mum and dad's first, then to Paul's parents for Christmas dinner, then back again to my parents' in the evening. I'd said to the girls at work that I'd like to get that all out of the way before I even thought about the baby's arrival. My dad always does a nice curry buffet on Christmas Day and I wanted to enjoy that first, then I'd be happy to have the baby any time afterwards.

Once Paul and I had given each other our own gifts at home, we stopped at my mum's about 12 noon. When I look back, I was wearing a bizarre outfit for someone who was nine months pregnant. I had thigh-length, high-heeled boots in brown leather that I'd folded down to my knees, black fishnet tights on, a ra-ra miniskirt and a tight brown top with a cowl neck. It was hardly maternity wear but I was still so slim that it seemed fine at the time. I didn't tell my parents I'd been feeling a bit strange; at that stage I hadn't put two and two together myself.

At about 2pm, we went to Alan and Kristina's for our Christmas lunch. There were nine or ten of us round the table. I kept feeling a strange pulling sensation, not a pain exactly, but it was odd. I didn't think to time it, but it was probably happening roughly every 20 minutes. By about 4pm, I was sitting in an armchair trying not to let anybody see that I was in discomfort, when Paul decided it would be a great idea to play a practical joke on his mum and Auntie Teresa by telling them that my waters had broken. He ran into the kitchen, practically flying through the door, shouting: 'Lindsey's waters have broken! Lindsey's waters have broken!' They all came screaming through and I said: 'No, he's joking!' – but all the time the pulling sensations were getting stronger.

Next time I got up from the chair I felt a bit funny. Paul's cousin Joanne asked me whether I was all right – I must have looked a bit odd – and I said: 'I just keep getting these funny pains, Joanne. It's like cramp.' Straight away she said, 'Linz! You're in labour!' I said, 'No! Course I'm not.' I think I was in denial. You wait for nine months, then think, 'God, no! I'm not having this. I'm not ready.'

The cramps got stronger but I was getting used to them and I thought to myself, Anyway, this could go on for days. Paul had drunk quite a bit by this stage and we needed to get to my parents, so I didn't really have much choice but to drive us there. We got in the car about 5.30pm and Joanne came out just as I was climbing in to the driver's seat. She asked me again if I was all right, and I had to catch my breath before I answered. 'I can't drive off quite yet, Joanne,' I said. 'Give me a minute.' 'Linz!' she said, 'I've said it already – you're in labour. You can't go driving around.' I told her I'd be absolutely fine and that I was sure it would wear off. I just wanted Paul to have a lovely Christmas Day. It wasn't often that he managed to get drunk by then and I wanted him to be able to carry on drinking and enjoying himself.

We got to my mum's about 6pm, and Paul went straight to their bar to help himself. Tracy and Chris were there with their kids, Matthew and Eloise, and my dad had the curry on the go. I went straight to Tracy and pulled her to the side. 'Trace,' I said, 'I just don't feel right.' I told her what had been going on and she echoed what Joanne had said – that I was in labour. Still I denied it. I couldn't be in labour, I just couldn't. She tried a different tack. 'All right then,' she said. 'Has there been anything else? Any trickles or shows?' I felt in a strong position this time. 'Absolutely not!' I said. 'Nothing at all.' The words were barely out of my mouth when it hit me. 'Oh God, Trace,' I said. 'Yesterday.' She stared at me. 'Yesterday what, our Linz? What are you talking about?' I told her that I'd felt fine but that I did think that I'd weed myself a lot because my pants kept getting wet. She said: 'Lindsey! They were wet because your waters were breaking! Why don't you just ring the delivery suite at the hospital and tell them what's been happening?'

I said that I would but asked Tracy not to tell Paul just yet. I'd been joking around with him, saying, 'Here Paul – the baby's on its way,' but he thought I meant in the next few days, not hours! I didn't want to panic him or get his hopes up if it was going to take ages. I'd had my bag packed and in the back of the car for ages, so I was ready to go. I phoned the delivery suite and said I was getting pains every 20 minutes. The midwife asked if the cramps were getting stronger, and I told her that when they were there I couldn't have a conversation or do anything but I was basically all right. She asked what colour the water was when it first came out, but I wasn't sure; I hadn't paid much attention to it but I thought it was clear like pee. She said that they needed to know if the baby has done a poo inside, and she warned me that these contractions could go on for a while. She said I could come down to the hospital if I wanted, but I was keener to stay at home as long as possible. I said that I'd wait until I had no choice, so we all tried to carry on as normally as possible. Tracy and I were the only ones who knew just what was going on.

We had our curry and then I suggested, 'Why don't we all have a game of Monopoly?' I've no idea why I said it because we hadn't done anything like that for years, but Chris and Tracy said they'd play with Paul and me. It was about 7pm by then, and I was just breathing and concentrating every time I got a cramp. Sometimes it got pretty sore and I'd say to Tracy, 'Can you move my counter for me?' Paul was oblivious. He was shouting, 'Pauline, large vodka and orange through here!' and I'd tell her, 'Make it a small one, Mum,' because although I still wanted him to have a nice time, I also wanted him to be able to come with me if the baby did arrive that night.

Paul was getting more and more drunk and I was getting more and more convinced that we had a heavy night ahead of us. 'What are we going to do if I'm too far gone to drive?' I asked Tracy. 'Stay here at Mum's,' she said, 'Then I can drive you to the hospital – or come back to mine and I'll look after you there.' Just as she said it, I felt odd again. I rushed out to the car and got a sanitary pad so that if anything did come out, I could tell the midwife what colour it was. I popped it in my knickers and then went back to playing Monopoly.

We were there for about an hour with the pains getting stronger. I never win anything so I wasn't too bothered about the game but Tracy and Chris usually enjoy being competitive. At about 8.30pm, I was getting bored so I suggested we just count up what money and property we had and call it a night. It turned out that I had won and Chris had come last – which never happens. Paul was laughing his head off, he was so drunk and happy. It was a miracle that I'd won, so I threw my arms up in the air and shouted, 'Yeah!' Straight away, my waters just came whoosh, flooding out onto the chair. You could actually hear them. Everyone shouted, 'What was that?' and it was absolute chaos in the room. I couldn't deny it this time – it was real. We were going to have a Christmas baby!

Chapter Thirty

Hello, Evie Rose

26 December 2005

I went to the toilet and could feel all this warm water soaking me. The moment I took my tights down, the pad fell down the loo and straight away the pains started to get stronger. I shouted to Tracy that I needed to go to the hospital without any delay. She was flapping about and her kids were screaming with excitement and Mum was shoving towels at me to put between my legs. 'Put your drink down, Paul! We're going!' I called. 'No chance,' he shouted, 'I need to calm my nerves so I'm having another!' Tracy got me into their Jeep. 'Where's Paul?' I asked her. 'He's out in the street, shouting "We're having a baby! My wife's having a baby!" like no one's ever done it before,' she told me.

Chris shoved him into the car and we drove to hospital. We knew the place inside out by now because of Paul's treatments but this time was different – this time we were there for something wonderful to happen. Tracy was laughing at me as I climbed out of the car. 'They're not going to think you're the one in labour. I'm the one wearing comfy clothes and you're in high heels and fishnets!' There were five flights of steps to climb, and I had to keep stopping and getting Paul and Tracy to wait for me to get my breath back. Meanwhile, Paul was still screaming, 'My wife's having a baby!'

On the ward they were very calm and nice. They told me to go into the assessment room and take my tights and boots off. As I got there, they wheeled out a woman with a baby, and Paul started crying. 'That's going to be us soon,' he was saying. 'Give me a chance, Paul,' I told him, 'I haven't done it yet.' He got a bit panicky when he saw me moaning in pain because I was usually the one in control. I had to reassure him between contractions that I was really OK. I asked Tracy to stay to keep us company, and also to help keep Paul calm.

The midwife came in to examine me and I could hardly believe it when she said I was only 2cm dilated. 'I don't think your waters have broken yet,' she stated calmly. I could have screamed at her! 'Believe me, they have,' I said. 'I needed wellies! I could have wrung my boots out there was so much.' She did a smear to check and said it looked a bit like mucus, but she wasn't sure. I was trying to stay calm but I was in pain and felt as though she wasn't listening to me. I said: 'I'm telling you, my waters have broken. It was all over the place.' She wasn't having any of it – I was told to go back downstairs and have a walk round the café to see if it might bring me on a bit. All she gave me for the pain were two bloody paracetamols!

I finally got down the steps to the café but it was horrendous. Paul was counting for me and the pains were coming every minute and a half. I went back and the midwife said it might stay like that for a while. By that time she agreed that my waters had broken but was still saying that I was hardly dilated at all. She asked me if I wanted to stay or go home, and I decided to go back to my mum's. I thought I'd be more relaxed there. Mum had a wheat bag that you could pop in the microwave and then place on your back and I thought it might provide more pain relief than a couple of paracetamols. The midwife assured me that I had ages to go, but she said if things hadn't progressed at all by morning then I would have to be induced as we'd need to get a move on now my waters had gone.

When we got to Mum's about 11pm, Chris was the only one awake. Mum had conked out on the sofa. Paul was clearly getting edgy and said that we should all have a drink. I tried to get him to agree that tea would be a good idea, but he wanted something stronger to calm his nerves. I decided I'd get in the bath to see if that would help ease the pain. Mum woke up and came to help me; I remember she was splashing water on my hair and face but I can't remember why because I got a bit delirious with the pain at times. She helped me get dried and gave me an old grey winceyette nightie of hers, which buttoned all the way up to the neck – it was a bit grim-looking but comfy. I got into my old childhood bed, but the pain was getting too much to bear and I soon realized that I needed to get back to the hospital, if only to get some proper pain relief.

I pulled some lilac velour trackie bottoms under the nightie and we got back in the Jeep. Paul brought his drink with him. I was wailing in agony all the way back into town.

About three miles from the hospital, I was lying back on the seat with my eyes shut. I was afraid that the baby was going to come out there and then, the pain was so bad. All of a sudden, I could feel the car slowing down. I knew we weren't there yet, because we hadn't been driving for long enough. I opened my eyes and right in front of us were five geese waddling across the dual carriageway really slowly. We weren't anywhere near a place that kept geese, and Paul and Tracy were in fits of hysterical laughter. I thought, 'Oh my God, I'm hallucinating. These two are laughing their heads off and singing about geese while I'm going to give birth!'

Finally, the geese did their thing and we headed off. Tracy parked and we were at the foot of those bloody stairs again. I'd hardly been away. Up at the ward, when I took my trackie bottoms off, there was blood absolutely everywhere. I thought something must have gone wrong but the midwife assured me that it was quite normal. She checked the baby's heartbeat and said that I'd gone up to 5cm dilated so I needed to go to the delivery room. I jumped off the bed and said, 'Fine. Where do you want me?' I was ready to get started and I didn't want any more delays. She tried to get me in a wheelchair, but I said I'd rather walk, so I hobbled into the delivery room and got up on the bed.

Paul and Tracy sat on chairs on either side of me. I took some gas and air but it made my mouth really dry so Paul kept going to get water for me and putting Vaseline on my lips. I dropped off into a kind of half sleep between contractions, but I had an odd feeling that everything was still going on and that it was getting close. Tracy was fantastic; I couldn't have done it without her. Paul spent his time reclining in a chair, pacing around, or going outside to smoke.

I don't often swear but I know I kept saying, 'Jesus Christ! Hail Mary!' and by the time it got to about 4am, I was ready to give in. I said to Tracy, 'I don't think I can do it any more. I'm so tired. I think I'm going to have to get something else because this gas and air isn't doing the job.' It must have been, though, because I was getting through it. Every time the midwife came in to check the baby's heartbeat, it was getting further down so I knew it was on the way. I could actually feel the bump moving downwards.

All of a sudden, I needed to push straight away. The midwife checked and said I was 10cm dilated so I could get on with it. I said, 'Honest? Is that it?' and she just smiled, and said that the baby was coming. I'd expected her to say that I couldn't push, that I wasn't allowed, but she told me to grab hold of my thighs and push as hard as I could. I remember this horrific stinging and I think I made a bit of noise. The midwife said the head would be out soon, so Tracy and Paul went down to have a look. The head came out with just one push and the midwife said it would only take one more after that to get the body out too. I could see my tummy going down in waves. As soon as the body came out, I just breathed a sigh of relief.

I was so stunned that I didn't even think to ask the big question. I heard the words, 'You've got a little girl,' and they didn't quite register. I said: 'It's a girl? Really? Are you sure?' I couldn't get my head round it. The midwife put the baby in my arms and the first thing I thought was, My God, she's purple. Incredibly purple. I asked if she was all right and the midwife said it was quite normal and she'd change in a couple of minutes. Paul was asked, 'Does Dad want to cut the cord?' and he hummed about a bit saying he wasn't sure, he didn't think he could do it, but he eventually took the scissors and did it. They clamped the baby and took her away for a check. I could hear the midwife say, 'Oooh, where did she get her red hair from?' but I was still shocked, and still asking if they were sure it was a girl!

When they told me that she weighed 6lbs 5oz, as Paul had predicted, I thought it was a joke. 'What did I tell you?' he shouted. 'I said I was having a girl, and I said she would be 6lbs 5oz.' How he knew that, I will never know.

She was brought back to us in a little towel. It was just the most bizarre thing. I still had to have an injection in my leg to get the placenta out but I didn't feel anything. Paul went from being very squeamish to saying that he'd like to see it! He was so proud. He said he didn't want to hold the baby when anybody else was in the room in case he didn't do it properly, but as soon as we were alone he took this tiny creature in his arms and kept saying over and over again, 'She's gorgeous, she's gorgeous.'

I looked at him, holding this little bit of life that we had made together, and it was just a perfect moment. In the middle of all the darkness and fear of death, all the pain and worry, we had created a new life.

'Paul,' I whispered, putting my arms around him as he held her so gently. 'That's our little girl. That's our Evie Rose.'

Chapter Thirty-one

A perfect family

26–31 December 2005

I couldn't believe what we had just done.

It was all so straightforward but incredible at the same time. Evie Rose had caught me a bit with her little fingernail on the way out but otherwise I didn't have any cuts or tears. Tracy had told me that you get a cup of tea and a plate of toast afterwards that is just the nicest in the world, and she was right. Evie was placed in a little sort of glass box at the side of us while my sister nipped out to ring our parents. Dad answered and he was just over the moon. Paul then rang his parents' house and told Leanne – we could hear them all screaming in the background.

A nurse turned the lights down so it was dark and cosy and so nice in the room. I lay in bed with Paul sitting in a chair beside me and we kept saying to each other, 'Can you believe that we've got a little girl?' The more we looked at her, the more real she seemed. Paul and I tried to shut our eyes but we couldn't get any sleep; we were so high on the whole experience. I got my mobile out and texted everyone in my phone book. I rang Nicky around 9am and shouted, 'I've got a little girl!' She was so happy for us. I texted everyone else to say: 'Hope u had a nice xmas day; I've got a little girl.' No one could believe I was on my mobile so soon after childbirth but I didn't want to go to sleep so I had to find something to occupy me.

The doctor had said that I could go home after six hours if everything was fine, so Tracy went back to our house to get the baby's car seat and fresh clothes and some bottles of formula. I decided to stick with my decision not to breastfeed because I guessed things were probably going to get tricky with Paul again and I might need to leave Evie with babysitters so I could be with him.

The midwife came in and said I could have a bath if I wanted and it was lovely to get washed and feel nice and clean again. I wasn't very sore at all – in fact, I felt normal and I was able to see my legs for the first time in ages. My bump had gone and I just felt a bit blubbery in my tummy. I could pick the skin up and wobble it back again in a way that was really quite horrible.

I put a tracksuit on but I didn't want to go back to the main ward because we were in this lovely safe little cocoon – just me, Paul and Evie Rose. Nothing could touch us in there. I couldn't wait to show her off to the world, but I knew that once we left that room, it would be back to real life and not knowing what the future was going to hold for Paul. Whatever it was going to be, he would now face it as a daddy.

I dressed Evie Rose all in white – we'd played it safe since we hadn't known the sex. The doctor came round and flicked the lights back to bright and I felt as if that was the end of that part, the end of our cocoon. I don't really pray, but I started to pray while the doctor did all the checks on her. I was just saying over and over again in my head: 'Please don't tell me there's anything wrong with her.' I didn't think I could bear it. The doctor was feeling down Evie's thighs; she looked so tiny without her nappy on, and he was pulling her legs and pushing her hips apart. I wanted to scream at him to be careful, and I was getting more and more worried the longer it went on. As if it was nothing, he casually mentioned that her left hip was a bit 'clicky'. I'd had a friend whose baby was 'clicky' and it turned out that her hip was dislocated and the baby had had to wear a hip brace for ages. I panicked a bit but the doctor said it might clear up on its own and they'd just keep an eye on it.

By then I wanted to get out of there and get her home where I could cuddle her all day. Paul said he felt a bit weird being in that hospital too; we had often gone past levels 4 and 5, which were the maternity wards, when he came in for chemo. We had seen people with their babies and thought that would be us one day – and now it was. We were leaving here with our own baby and that was such a wonderful thing that I could put clicky hips and cancer and everything negative out of my head for a while at least.

Chris and Tracy came back with the car seat. As it was winter, we'd bought a cream snowsuit for the baby to go home in. It had looked tiny in the shop but when we put Evie in it, you could hardly even see her. There was just her tiny little head poking out. She wasn't jaundiced but she looked really brown – in fact, in all her pictures she looked tanned for weeks. Paul was carrying her, the very picture of a proud dad, and I was hobbling to the car. I wasn't in pain exactly – you just put that to the back of your mind – but I was uncomfortable; every bump in the road felt sore. Chris said: 'I can't believe you're going home. Tracy was in hospital for more than a week with Matthew. Are you trying to set a record? We were only playing Monopoly just over 12 hours ago, and now you're back in the car with a baby.' I noticed that he didn't mention me winning, so things were back to normal.

Paul hadn't had anything to drink for a while now, so he was sober. I wanted to go to my mum and dad's straight away. We got there and I popped Evie on their breakfast bar in her car seat. It was about 12.30pm on Boxing Day and it didn't seem like Christmas any more. Normally one of us would be having a party but instead we were looking at Evie, all of us standing there together.

My aunt Pauline came round to have a look (and a cry!), then we decided to get off home. I sat in the back seat again so that I could look at Evie the whole time. I just wanted to stare at her.

Tracy had organized everything perfectly back at ours, but I was a bit dazed and didn't know what to do once she had left. It was just us on our own and we didn't have any experience of babies. I'd tried to give Evie a bottle in the hospital and she didn't seem to want it. The midwife said she was probably tired and might not want much, but I felt that she should be getting fed. Nicky had lent us a Moses basket, so I put her in that because she'd been in the car seat for a while and I worried that her spine would get too curved. She was beautiful; so relaxed. Paul sat on the sofa and I put the fire on and we both just looked at our baby for ages. She only filled about a quarter of the Moses basket.

After a while, we felt as though we should do something, so we got out the nappies, cotton wool, bottles, all the stuff we needed, and waited for her to wake up. Then, while we were waiting, we both dozed off to sleep. I woke up with a start and got in such a panic. 'Paul!' I screamed, 'I've been asleep! How could I have gone to sleep when there's no one else to look after the baby?' Paul woke up properly and said: 'It's probably all right. She seems fine. How about we have a go at changing her bum? Let me do it.'

We laid the changing mat by the fire where it was all cosy. What a performance it all was to begin with! I was in charge of getting the warm water in a bowl, and standing by with the cotton wool balls and the clean nappy. I'd done it before with Matthew and Eloise and some friends' babies, but Paul was a novice. Evie had only had a teensy bit of milk so I thought it would be an easy one for him to get started on – but when we opened up the nappy there was black sticky poo all over her. Paul was panicking because it was stuck to her bum and then she was sick and he became frantic.

'I don't believe it!' he shouted. 'My first time, and this all happens at once! How can such a little thing have so much coming out of her? The poo's welded to her backside like cement!' I reassured him that it was all fine, and we both tackled Evie together. It took the two of us working side by side and we were exhausted by the time she had a clean nappy on, but it was hilarious at the same time, and lovely to be sharing this experience.

I really miss that now – the sharing, the being together doing perfectly normal stuff but feeling that it's special because you're together in your own little world.

After the nappy change, I called Tracy, worried that Evie still wasn't really taking any milk. Tracy said it was fine and she might not take anything till the next day; she would eat when she was ready. Paul was shouting in the background, 'How can she have so much coming out at both ends then?'

We spent most of the afternoon just looking at her. It is such an incredible thing to look at your own baby; it doesn't matter how many other babies you've seen, your own just blows you away. For Paul, it was one of the happiest moments of his life. He'd always wanted a daughter – I remember him saying to Nicky's and Tracy's husbands that they were so lucky they had girls. He often said: 'A son would be great, but it takes a real man to have a daughter.' I don't know where he got that from, or what he was on about really, but he seemed to have this need to be a daddy to a little girl.

At about 6pm, Kris and Alan came over with Paul's Aunt Teresa and Grandma Babcia. They all looked at the baby and had a cuddle and took a million pictures, saying that it was amazing to think she wasn't much more than 12 hours old. Looking back, the main thing I remember is how tiny she was and how the happiness was just bursting out of Paul. We hadn't spoken about cancer in the middle of all this, of course, and we never allowed it to creep in and spoil things. When you look at the man you love and the baby you both love, together, wrapped up in each other, it would probably break your heart to even imagine for a second that it might all come to an end soon. Those early moments were so magical – but mostly for me, I suppose, given that Paul isn't here to know what he's missing, and Evie won't remember the first cuddle with her dad, the first kiss, or the dozens of other firsts he had with his little girl.

Paul's family left after a couple of hours and it hit us that we were shattered. I hadn't really slept since I'd given birth, not properly, and Paul was dealing with the exhaustion of being ill on top of everything else. We needed to sleep desperately but we weren't sure that it was safe to leave her unsupervised. It seemed reckless not to be watching her constantly. We put the Moses basket next to my side of the bed, but didn't dare sleep for ages. She woke up about twice in the night but just made these little noises, little puffy whispers. Paul leapt straight up for cotton wool and hot water and a warm bottle of milk, as if she had screamed the house down. I got her changed and we sat there cuddling her and cooing.

Next morning we carried her downstairs in her basket, still sleeping. That first day set the pattern. We just did everything together for the first week. Your life is full of nothing but your baby and it's the most wonderful thing in the world. I'm not one for lounging about, but I did more of it that first week than I've ever done and it was the nicest week of my life. If I could get that week back, I'd be the happiest person in the world. We were in the house every day more or less. I think I only nipped out twice for milk. There was a constant stream of visitors, so I'd get everyone to bring whatever we needed with them.

Evie was so easy to look after for the first few days, just sleeping and feeding; I suppose she was getting over the trauma of the birth. She was only taking an ounce of milk at a time then sleeping for four hours straight. She was still so little. We took a picture of her next to the TV remote control to show how tiny she was. Every day we'd choose a new little babygro for her to wear. Her wardrobe was just crammed with outfits; she was spoiled from the start. We got into a routine of napping on the sofa while she was asleep, and waking when she was awake. It was a great time to have Evie, while Paul was between treatments, because it meant he could bathe her and feed her and get to know her without feeling ill all the time. I was on a high.

On New Year's Eve Tracy invited us over to her house. We seemed to have to fill the car to breaking point just to spend one night away from home: we took the sterilizer, the Moses basket, baby monitors, bottles, about a dozen changes of clothes, bedding, cotton wool, nappies and a million other things! I dressed Evie in a lovely little pink dress and only had time to have a quick shower myself and run my fingers through my hair.

Paul was drinking that night, and I had a few drinks myself. It was strange – we were happy but emotional as the clock moved towards midnight. Paul had a bit of a cry. 'God, Lindsey,' he kept saying. 'What a year. What a year. I've felt so poorly and there were times I thought I was going to die, but now I've never been happier. I've got a baby!' I shed a few tears as well, which isn't like me. 'I know, darling,' I said, 'We've got Evie Rose, and maybe things will go right for us now.' I was trying to inject a bit of optimism into him, but he turned to me and said, 'You know what? It doesn't matter. I'm not really bothered what happens now.' I told him not to be so daft, to stop saying silly things, but there was a chill going up my spine. He wouldn't stop. 'I've brought someone into this world, so I don't care about myself. I've done something. We've done something together.' I told him not to say such things, that we had a lovely future ahead of us watching Evie grow up. He didn't say anything else; he just sort of went into himself for a bit.

Paul wasn't the only one reflecting on what 2005 had brought us. My mum was crying her eyes out, saying, 'Oh, what a year they've had, what a year.' Someone else said that it had all ended well and we had Evie so things must be looking up. Paul seemed to be getting back to himself after a while, and we all stood out on Tracy's deck where there was a view for miles. He stayed out there on his own after the rest of us came in and I worried that he was thinking negative thoughts again.

He came in after a while and said, 'Tracy, I've got good news and bad news. The good news is that I've got room for another drink. The bad news is that I've been sick over your terrace onto someone's car!' He said that he was so used to being sick from the chemo that it made a nice change for it to be happening because of the booze. He seemed to be back to his old self again, but I couldn't help wondering about what he'd said earlier. Were these the sorts of thoughts he pondered by himself, things he usually chose not to share with me?

Now I wonder why I didn't set more store by it – he'd been right about so many other things. Maybe he was trying to warn me about what was next in line for us. It didn't matter how bad my mum thought 2005 had been – it would soon seem like a picnic compared to 2006.

Chapter Thirty-two

Wishing for miracles

January–March 2006

Three days after the New Year's Eve party at Tracy's, on 3 January, Paul had an appointment with Dr Chester at the hospital to discuss what to do next. He was straight with us, as he'd always been.

'Paul, I'm afraid the chemotherapy isn't working any more. It's keeping your tumour marker level stable but not reducing it, so I don't think there's any point in doing another cycle at the moment.'

'What will we do instead?' I asked straight away, my throat feeling tight.

He seemed embarrassed. 'Let's just keep taking the medication for the next few weeks and keep an eye on things. Your body's had quite enough chemo to deal with over the last year. Go home, have a rest and we'll have a think about what to do next.'

Paul and I looked at each other, but neither of us asked the questions that were going through our heads. If they weren't treating him any more, did that mean he was going to die?

And if so, how much time did he have left? There's no way we could have asked these questions, but I think from this consultation onwards, both of us were privately starting to wonder.

Dr Chester did his best to put a positive spin on it, but I came away from the meeting alarmed that the medical profession seemed to be scratching their heads. Basically, they didn't know what to do next. I decided I was going to have to take matters into my own hands and do all the research I could about alternative treatments and lifestyle changes that might help.

Paul was very quiet on the way home. He seemed a bit dazed, a bit lost, but very relieved not to be facing the next cycle of chemo straight away. He could spend some quality time with our daughter and play some snooker without feeling so ill all the time. Paul had utter faith in his doctors throughout the treatment. He believed they were all doing the best for him that they possibly could and after 3 January, he clung to the hope that a new wonder drug would come out any day. I wasn't quite so optimistic. I reckoned that if there were any other options out there, it was up to me to find them and make sure he got every possible chance.

Because Paul was in the public eye, his diagnosis and progress had been reported in the media. Along with all the good luck and get well messages, letters and cards, there were lots of people who got in touch suggesting remedies that Paul should try. I honestly think that the vast majority of them came from people who had Paul's best interests at heart. I know that there are probably some organizations out there who profit from other people's misery but either Brandon screened us from them or we were very lucky.

Amongst other messages we got through Brandon, there was one from Steve Davis, the snooker player, who told us that a relative of his had been diagnosed with cancer a little while ago and he had used essiac tea to help cure him. I looked into this and found that it was a herbal recipe that had been discovered over 70 years ago by a Canadian nurse. She had been told about it by a breast cancer patient who had been given it by a Native American medicine man. This woman allegedly recovered from her breast cancer and lived another 30 years with no recurrence of the cancer. The nurse used the same recipe on her aunt, who had terminal stomach and liver cancer – and she lived another 21 years. After this, the nurse set up her own clinic in Canada providing essiac tea to anyone who came to consult her. She went into a research partnership with one of John F. Kennedy's physicians and treated hundreds of people over the years.

Essiac tea had apparently helped patients with AIDS, diabetes, asthma, Parkinson's disease and Alzheimer's, as well as cancer. Of course, you never know whether it was the tea that worked or something else – but the fact that we knew someone who said that a member of their family had been helped by it made me think that Paul should give it a try. Paul was sceptical – but I was desperate.

We bought a few packets and made it up according to the instructions. It sounded pretty straightforward and innocuous. The tea is made from burdock root, sheep sorrel, turkey rhubarb root and slippery elm bark. That meant nothing to me, but the fact that it was all natural and organic had to be good, given that Paul's body had been subjected to so much that wasn't remotely natural. I had to sterilize everything and fill a stainless steel pan with spring water that had no sodium in it. Then I put the tea in, stirred and boiled it again for 10 minutes. It was left to stand for six hours with a cover on it, the cover was lifted, it was stirred and left for another six hours. It was then reheated to boiling point and strained into another sterilized stainless steel pan, before I cleaned the original pan and strained the tea back into that. Then it was poured into eight sterilized glass bottles and stored. I felt as though I was brewing up a witches' potion! It took ages, but at least I was doing something instead of just sitting back to see what would happen.

It smelled horrible when I poured out the first cup and passed it to Paul. It had barely touched his lips before he spat it out again.

'Christ, Lindsey!' he said. 'What the hell is that? Are you trying to poison me now?'

I tried to encourage him. 'Now come on, Paul,' I said. 'It's good for you.'

'How d'you know that then?' he asked. 'Tastes like it'll kill me straight away.'

Bless him – he did try, and I did keep making it up for him, but he hated it and could barely get any of it down.

When you first hear of things like that, you might be a bit sceptical, but there is such desperation for something, anything that might do the trick that you end up thinking, Well, why not? Maybe it will be the miracle we're hoping for. All the clinical approaches had been tried and things were as bad as ever – worse – so why not think there might be something else? The cynicism goes and you get a bit of hope. It's odd, though; I found the hope got blown away as soon as there was a bit of resistance – so, as soon as Paul said he didn't like essiac tea and was fed up having to drink it, I immediately thought, Ah well, it's probably a load of old rubbish, anyway.

That's the cycle you go through.

Until the next idea.

We tried a couple of other remedies and then, in February 2006, Brandon was contacted by a couple who ran an alternative health practice in Cornwall. This man – Alex – said in his letter: 'I read about Paul's fight against cancer recently and as someone with a young family myself, I was drawn to do what I can to help.' He wasn't asking for anything, he didn't want money or to make us buy some wonder drug; he just wanted to give Paul some information. Alex had been putting together an information booklet for his clients about the factors that affect good health and well-being. He said that he wanted to make sure Paul was as informed as possible and that all avenues for his recovery were being explored. I couldn't argue with that – it was what we all wanted.

Alex said that conventional medicine often seemed to overlook many simple and obvious causes of cancer, and didn't link many of the causes together. He said that it was important that Paul's bodily imbalances were detected and corrected, so that his body would have the best chance of healing itself naturally. As far as I was concerned, if there was a single shred of hope out there, the slightest possibility that we had missed something, I was ready to grab it.

Alex told us that there were three main causes of imbalance which Paul should be aware of – it was then up to him whether he wanted to take it further and investigate whether any of them related to him. The first one was parasites. Alex said that these were at epidemic proportions in the Western world and caused lots of serious illness – including cancer. He said that creatures like tapeworms could live in our intestines for years without us having any notion that they were ever there. All the while they would be preventing us absorbing the vitamins and minerals our bodies needed, making us weak. What a thought!

The second problem could be geopathic stress. I'd never heard of this but Alex said it had been found to be a common factor in most serious, long-term illnesses and psychological conditions – again, including cancer. He explained that geopathic stress is a kind of natural radiation, which rises up through the earth and is distorted by weak electromagnetic fields. These fields are created by subterranean running water, certain mineral concentrations, fault lines and underground cavities. Blimey – I'd certainly never thought of any of that being a cause of illness. He went on to say that the wavelengths of natural radiation disturbed by phenomena can actually become harmful to living organisms – the immune system can be affected. I felt myself squirming as he explained this. Alex continued by saying that geopathic stress needs to be blocked 100 per cent for the immune system to work properly. Apparently, research showed that

85 per cent of people suffering ill health are sleeping in geopathic stress areas, although conventional medicine never gives this a second thought.

The final factor he said we needed to be aware of was electromagnetic stress. This is mainly caused by electrical appliances – TVs, computers, microwaves, mobiles and suchlike, as well as railway lines, pylons, power stations and so forth. Electromagnetic stress can have the same effect as geopathic stress, possibly in an even stronger and more damaging way.

It all sounded promising. If any of these things were affecting Paul, it was easy to see that they could cause serious illness. Alex didn't ask for anything; he just sent us some photocopied articles and said we could find out about it all online if we did a quick search. I did – and I knew that I wanted to talk to him. When we spoke on the phone, he suggested that I send him some of Paul's nail clippings, which he could test to see if any of the factors he had mentioned were relevant. Also, if I drew a plan of the ground floor of our house, he could ask someone who knew a bit about geopathic and electromagnetic stress to take a look at it. If we wanted to buy a device that would block harmful radiation, he could put us in touch with someone. I know that for some people, the warning lights would already be flashing – but I didn't feel that way, and nothing proved me wrong. The blocker and nail clipping tests cost less than £200 – and I don't see how anyone could make their fortune out of that!

I drew a quick plan of the ground floor of our house and sent off the nail samples. I put in a note to say that Paul's nails were very brittle due to the chemotherapy. The results came back quickly, by the last week in February. The report said that Paul was being severely affected by geopathic stress, and that he had a tapeworm we needed to get rid of. He had a high level of emotional stress (unsurprisingly!) and there were traces of toxic metals in his body – from fillings, paint fumes, lead petrol and suchlike – that needed to be flushed out. His main organs weren't functioning properly – again, unsurprisingly – and his immune system was sluggish. Some of this could easily have been guessed, given that everyone knew he had cancer and had been undergoing chemo, but I was willing to give Alex's suggestions a try.

I bought a 'blocker' for the geopathic stress and was told where to place it in the lounge. To get rid of the tapeworm, Paul needed to take a homeopathic remedy twice a day for five weeks. A nutritional yeast product would help to transport oxygen around Paul's body and he was to stick to a strict vegan diet for four months – no dairy, fish, eggs or meat. I could see that would be a big problem for Paul – he liked his bacon sarnies dripping in butter. There were other suggestions about certain natural remedies to try, and I was willing to give them all a go. I didn't see how any of it could harm him and it might just help.

Paul was happy to try it out, but I must say that he never committed to the programme 100 per cent. He still wanted to smoke, and drink when he could, and, because his appetite was so poor, it was hard for him to be on a restricted diet. Also, he was smoking quite a lot of joints as those helped to stimulate his appetite. I was a bit upset that he didn't go for it completely, but it was his body, his choice – I would never push him too far.

In the midst of all this, we had some good news. At the end of February it was time for Evie to get her hips checked to see if she would need to wear a hip brace. I was panicking, thinking, Please don't give me the trauma of coming back to the hospital with Evie as well as Paul. I remember feeling the nerves in my tummy. I took her to the same place we'd gone to for the antenatal scans and Leanne came with us. I was muttering, 'Please, please, please,' to myself just as I had done the first time she was examined. A nurse came in, undressed her and placed her between two cushions. They did an ultrasound and finally the nurse said that the hip was still a little bit clicky, but it was within the normal range so she should be fine.

I was overwhelmed with relief. It felt like a real break to be told something good at a hospital for once. I might be strong, but I wasn't sure that I'd have had enough strength to fight two battles at once.

As it was, I could turn my attention back to Paul again – and there was another possible miracle cure waiting for us round the corner. It was time for 'loony juice'.

Chapter Thirty-three

Father Christmas
April–June 2006

*P*aul felt much better in the months when he wasn't having chemo. I think at times he forgot how serious his cancer was. Living with it was much easier than treating it, and we still had a bit of faith in the teas and homeopathic remedies and geopathic blockers.

For this reason, Paul was very upset when Dr Chester suggested he do another cycle of chemotherapy that April. It was a different kind of chemo this time – oxaliplatin and capecitabine – but we both found it extremely depressing to go back into the old routine of driving there, having the blood tests done, hanging around, then the three days of drip-feeding and flushing out, followed by the horrendous nausea and vomiting. What's more, this new chemo sent his markers sky high, up to 150,000, which was unbelievably depressing.

Paul was still playing snooker as the 2005/6 season came to an end. At the Masters in February he had lost to Mark Williams in the first round, and had shocked everyone there with his puffed-up appearance, his bald head and grey-tinted skin. At what would turn out to be his last professional match, at the Crucible in April, he was beaten by Neil Robertson (a player Brandon now manages). Everyone there could see he was very poorly, a shadow of his former self, but he still hung around afterwards chatting to fans and signing autographs just as he had always done. The little boy whose ambition at the age of 10 had been to play at the Crucible moved everyone who saw him there that day, whether in the flesh or on the TV coverage.

Just as Paul was finishing his sixth cycle of chemo, Brandon told me about an Australian guy who had been in touch and wanted to talk about an unlicensed product that he claimed had been behind some amazing recovery stories. I was a bit suspicious, especially since the medicine was unlicensed, but we decided to take Paul to meet him and see what he had to offer.

It was like having an appointment with Father Christmas. The man behind this 'miracle cure' had a big white bushy beard and just seemed to exude warmth. I immediately felt calmed and convinced by him. Both Brandon and I signed confidentiality agreements about much of the information we were given, but there were some general points that 'Santa' was willing to discuss with anyone. He started by admitting that he had absolutely no medical background – in fact his background was in mining engineering. However, he and some friends had, by accident, discovered a compound that worked amazingly well in animals with cancer. They then worked with a team of doctors to develop the com-

nbreakable

pound and make it suitable for human use and had now treated a number of patients across the globe. Santa said that the results had been astounding – people who were on their last legs and who had given up all hope with conventional treatment had been in remission for years after taking this liquid.

My concern was still that it was unlicensed. Santa explained that the cancer drug market was big business for corporations and that he believed his product would never get approval since he was threatening the lucrative financial side of the business. If he had actually found a cure, what would that mean for the companies who produced drugs and treatments which only delayed death for a few months?

'I don't know, Paul,' I said. 'It sounds too good to be true – but what do you think?'

Paul had been taking everything in and asking lots of questions. Now he turned to me and said, 'Lindsey, I've tried it all. I've been blasted to kingdom come with chemo and the cancer keeps coming back. I'll try anything – especially if it's something that might take this bloody awful disease by surprise.'

Santa told us a bit more about the liquid, which I soon began to call 'loony juice'. Paul wouldn't just have to take it in measured doses a number of times a day; he would also have to completely clear his system. No booze, no fags, no drugs. He would also have to stop any conventional medical treatment. This meant there was a difficult decision to make. Was he willing to forego the next cycle of chemotherapy that he was due to start in a couple of weeks' time?

This was a huge decision and I wasn't at all sure what was

right, but after talking it through some more, Paul decided that, yes, he'd give it a try.

'Are you sure, babes?' I said to him. 'No one is pushing you into anything. I only want you to make decisions that you want to make.'

'I've felt that I haven't had any choices to make for months,' Paul said. 'I'm making this one.'

So that was that. When we told Dr Chester about his decision, he was very nice about it. He spoke to Father Christmas on the phone and then wrote to Paul to wish him well and assure him that he would be there at any stage if Paul wanted to go back to conventional treatments. He did say that the loony juice treatment couldn't be supported medically but he wished us luck with it.

Before he started the new regime, Paul decided to have one last fling. He and the boys went to Amsterdam at the end of April 2006 just to chill out in the cannabis cafés, smoking and drinking and having fun. I encouraged him to go because he needed to relax, and he deserved some sort of reward after what he had been through. He had a great time there and felt more like himself than he had for ages, just hanging out with the lads.

The day he got back it was time to start on Santa's regime. We were given lots and lots of instructions to follow. Before Paul could start taking the actual loony juice, he had to clear all the toxins from his body. He had to drink another solution that Santa supplied first. We were told that his body would get rid of all the waste in quite a dramatic way – and it did; he passed so much black poo that we thought something must be going horribly wrong. It was constant, and he felt terrible, but we were reassured that this was all part of the process and meant that the loony juice would be much more effective. Paul even stopped smoking, which was a huge commitment from him. I couldn't believe he finally managed it, but this was just another sign of the enormous faith we felt in loony juice at the outset.

The other commitment we made was a financial one – we spent £28,000 on loony juice altogether, but I never felt as though we were being duped; I honestly felt, as Paul did, that there was a chance this might work. I said to him at the time that the money didn't matter. If it looked as though it was working, the family would all sell our houses to keep him on it for as long as he needed.

Within a week of Paul starting to take the loony juice, he started to feel better. His appetite came back, he had the energy to do things like playing with Evie, taking her out to the park, and he had no pain.

'I feel fantastic!' he told me one morning. 'I feel as good as I felt 18 months ago before this all started.'

He continued to have a weekly blood test at St James' to get his cancer markers checked and before long, miraculously, the loony juice seemed to be working. His levels dropped from 150,000 down to 30,000 – still way too high but a huge improvement in such a short time.

But Paul felt so good that he started having the odd cigarette again. I think he forgot how bad the cancer was because he was feeling so great. On 24 June, we went to two weddings in the one day: his cousin Craig's in the afternoon, and then the evening do for his friends Ash and Jodie. It was the last day he felt well – and the last time a lot of friends saw him.

Because after that there was a setback. A big one. On 27 June, Paul woke in the morning feeling dreadful. He was clutching his side and moaning, 'Linz, the pain in my side. It's back. The tumour's getting bigger. I know it is.'

'You can't know that,' I said, panicking. 'We need to give the loony juice longer to work.'

'I do know, Linz. I know my own body. It's coming back. I just know it.'

The next blood test confirmed it: his markers were back up to 40,000. The loony juice had bought him six fantastic weeks when he felt absolutely wonderful, but in the end the cancer had just got too strong. We decided to stop paying for more loony juice at that stage and go back to conventional treatment again.

Looking back, I still think we were absolutely right to try the loony juice because it gave Paul those six good weeks in spring 2006. And at least we could be a hundred per cent sure that we had tried everything we could and left no stone unturned in looking for a cure.

Chapter Thirty-four

Summer 2006

*R*eality kicked in when he got his next test results through – things were going downhill, and the decline was much more rapid than any signs of recovery had ever been. Just as Paul had predicted, the next scan showed that his tumour had started to grow. No one could deny it any more. Paul was getting worse, almost by the day.

The doctors decided to treat him with another cycle of chemotherapy – but personally I really thought they were clutching at straws by now. I could see it in their expressions sometimes. They didn't pretend to be trying for a cure any more – they were just trying to stop the tumour getting any bigger.

We were fed up with the sight of St James' so we arranged that Paul could be treated at a private hospital called the Elland, in Halifax, which had lovely gardens and a more luxurious décor. It was also handier for the family to visit because you could park right outside. For this cycle of chemo, Paul was treated as a day patient and got to come home every night so long as he took the tablets at set times.

Paul had always been terrible at swallowing tablets, and these ones were massive. He needed to take five in the morning and five at night, so I crushed them up in yoghurt and fed them to him.

I was back at work part-time by now, trying to keep some semblance of normality in my life, so I asked Darren Clarke and Paul's cousin Anthony to come and stay for a while to keep Paul company when I wasn't there. In fact, as it turned out, they would both stay with us for the next few months and Anthony took some time out of college so he could continue to help.

The three of us made a good team: I gave Paul the love, Anthony tended to look after practical things like making sure he took his medication at the right times, and Daz was the one who could make him laugh!

Paul lost a lot of weight that summer and began to feel ill most of the time. The pain increased so much that, at times, he could barely lift his head from the sofa. He would lie around in a white towelling robe that he seemed to live in for months. Friends were shocked when they came to visit during July because he looked absolutely terrible. His abdomen was becoming rounded and so swollen that it looked as though he was pregnant. He couldn't sleep for more than an hour at a time and he spent most of the day and night propped up on the sofa or in a beanbag in the den. He was so sick that he had no appetite at all, even when I tried to tempt him with favourite foods like bacon sarnies. And his skin was grey and painful to the touch, so often I couldn't even give him a comforting hug.

He'd stopped taking the loony juice at the end of June when he felt the pain in his side return, but I persuaded him to go back on it again in August. I was desperate. I would have tried anything at all that I thought would help, no matter how weird or wacky others might think it was.

Of course, I was still trying to look after Evie at the same time and when Paul had a slightly better day, I'd get him to help – purely as a way of taking him out of himself. It may sound harsh, but there were days when I would put Evie down beside him and say, 'I'm popping out for a bit, Paul.' I'd only stand outside the front door, but I reasoned that, if he was forced to look after her, he would. It would take him a lot of effort to sit up and pick her up if she was whimpering, but when I came back in again, she'd be lying contentedly in his arms and he'd be so proud.

Paul enjoyed choosing Evie's clothes for the day. If he could get up, he would go and look in her wardrobe and say, 'Can you put this on her today, Linz?' He couldn't dress her himself because his fingers were so affected by the treatment that he found press studs and buttons impossible. Despite all his pain, he loved feeding her from a bottle and I was so glad I'd given him that option and not decided to breastfeed.

He just loved being a dad and I loved watching him holding her in his arms and looking at her with such love in his eyes. I wish now I had videoed them together but Paul wasn't keen because he looked so terrible that he didn't want any pictures taken. We've still got some lovely photos from Evie's first few months, though.

After that cycle of chemo, on 30 August we went to see the

doctors again and the message came back that Paul's markers were still shooting up. I knew by now that our options had pretty much run out unless there was such as thing as a miracle. The messages from the doctors were quite clear – where once they had spoken of a cure, then remission, then partial remission, they now only talked of symptom control, pain management and palliative care. He was so weak by this time that he couldn't have taken any more aggressive treatments, even if there had been anything left to try.

One Wednesday towards the end of August, Paul had to go to Cookridge for a CT scan and Darren went with him. St James' rang to ask if he could go in for a meeting afterwards, so the two of them went along to speak to Dr Chester. If I had known the question Paul would ask at that meeting, I would have made sure I was there but I don't think he had planned it himself; it just came out.

He asked, 'If there are no treatments left for me to try, how long have I got then?'

Dr Chester gave him a straight answer. 'If and when there are no more treatments left for us to try, you may get three months – six if you're lucky.' Lucky! What did luck have to do with any of this? What a ridiculous word to use in these circumstances.

All I knew was that my mobile phone rang and I heard Paul screaming on the other end, completely hysterical. 'They said I've only got six months left to live!'

I could hardly make out what he was saying, he was so upset.

'Go home, babes,' I said. 'I'll meet you there as soon as I can.'

Anthony drove me home, crying my eyes out, and when I got back I ran upstairs and found Paul sitting on the toilet. The fact that I was upset made him even more upset. 'I thought you'd be calm,' he cried. 'I thought you'd say "Don't be silly – it'll all be fine."'

We cried together for about 10 minutes and then I pulled myself together. I said, 'Up until the last treatment happens, you're still here – so let's be positive. If and when there are no more treatments left, then you've maybe only got six months. But you're still doing chemo and we're trying the loony juice, so we mustn't give up hope.'

Paul calmed down, but I knew in myself that his chances had run out. He probably wouldn't be there the following year. Would he make Christmas? I didn't know.

Paul was going to die – and it would be sooner rather than later.

Of course, being Paul, it wasn't long before he was making a joke out of it: 'Right lads!' he said to the boys when we went downstairs. 'We've got 5 months, 29 days and 12 hours left to have some fun!'

People still ask whether it was unbearable to watch him get closer to death every day, but I was seeing him constantly so I didn't actually notice the physical decline in a dramatic way. If friends hadn't been round for even as little as a week they would say how much worse he looked, but I didn't see it that way. He was still my Paul.

We told Kris and Alan what Dr Chester had said but they were still clinging to the hope that the latest treatments would work, or that a new miracle drug would be discovered. There was one time when I was with Nicky and I broke down and told her that I didn't think Paul would be around for Christmas, that he was disappearing before my eyes, but she wasn't ready to accept it. 'Come on, Linz,' she said. 'Whatever happened to your famous positive attitude?'

That summer we got a Macmillan nurse who started to come round, and she was an absolute blessing because she was able to reassure Paul about individual symptoms he was having and give him whatever he needed to deal with the pain. I remember them saying at one point that they should have allocated us a Macmillan nurse a lot earlier, and I think that would have been great. I almost don't know what to say about them – they are just so good, and so comforting. Paul always loved being at home, he'd do anything to get out of going to a hospitalized setting, so having a nurse coming to talk to him at home was so much better. Right up to the last days, if I ever suggested to him, 'Paul, you're in agony, we need to get to hospital now,' he'd always say, 'No way.' He preferred to wait till his Macmillan nurse got there so she could sort him out at home.

On 16 September, Cathy Douglas, a friend of Paul's who ran a company called Moor Fizz, had organized a big fundraising event called Paul Hunter's Big Night Out, at the Lido in Ilkley. Sadly, just before the day came, Paul was diagnosed as being dehydrated and there was no choice but to admit him to hospital for rehydration through a drip. I went on my own – I was getting used to standing in for him now – and my dad couldn't believe it when I took the microphone and started addressing the crowd. I hadn't done much public speaking before, apart from teaching beauty students, and ordinarily the thought would have terrified me – but it was such a good cause that I believed in wholeheartedly that all nerves just left me. I can't remember exactly what I said, but I was touched at how proud Dad was of me that day. The audience included tennis player Tim Henman, snooker players Stephen Hendry, Mark Williams, Matthew Stevens, John Virgo and Jimmy White. Alex Ferguson sent a personal message to Paul, saying for him to keep his chin up!

The auction that night raised a fortune for a charity in Paul's name to help others suffering from intestinal cancer. Paul had already donated £15,000 to it from the proceeds of a golf day run by Cantor Fitzgerald. I was chuffed to bits when, halfway through the evening, Paul texted me to tell me he was sure I'd be looking gorgeous!

When Paul got out of hospital that time, he couldn't eat solids any more and he was existing on protein drinks. All the same, he was sick constantly – 30 or 40 times in the space of a couple of days. When he was sick, he'd hand me the bowl and I'd go to the sink, wash it out and bring it back to him again. What more could I do? He was on morphine tablets and morphine patches but they did nothing but make him throw up even more. He walked slowly, hunched over with the pain in his abdomen. He couldn't sleep so Daz and Anthony took it in shifts, staying up all night with him to watch movies or get him whatever he needed. I didn't want him to be awake on his own in the middle of the night; that's the loneliest time.

We didn't really talk about any of it — we never did that; there was no point, you just have to get on with things. Paul knew that being well again was so far beyond what he could hope for that he had lowered his sights to wishing he could get just an hour of sleep. When he was doing badly I was helpless — there was nothing I could do. From the end of August, every single day was misery for him.

I knew our time together was limited, that every day was taking us closer to his final hours, but all I could do was be there for him. He fought so hard — I could sometimes hear him thrashing about in his sleep, saying things which were unintelligible but which sounded like a man fighting against something; something that we both knew the name of but never spoke of directly these days.

On Tuesday 3 October Paul had been sick all through the night and seemed dehydrated again. I had to go to work but I arranged for a Macmillan nurse to pop in that afternoon. As soon as she arrived, she said he had to get to hospital but Paul refused to go without seeing Evie and me first. I picked Evie up and drove home about 6pm, then we packed Paul's pillow and duvet and chocolate-brown throw into the car, as we always did when he was off to hospital.

We had no sense that this was the end; that this was the last time he would see his own house or watch telly in the den or play pool in the games room. As far as we were concerned, it was another routine trip to hospital for re-hydration and he'd be home in a few days' time. At about 7.30pm, Anthony drove Paul to the hospital; Paul was wearing his white robe and grey trackie pants underneath.

Next morning, I dropped Evie at my mum's first thing and went to the hospital to visit him. I got a huge shock when I walked into the room because for the first time Paul was in a wheelchair. That had never happened before. His eyes were sunken, his skin was pale and stretched over his face and somehow his teeth looked bigger in his skull. For the first time, he looked to me as though he was dying. Anthony was in tears outside the room.

I went to find a doctor, and although I could sense it was true, I was still gobsmacked at what he told me. 'I'm afraid there's nothing more we can do, Lindsey. It's time to get Paul to a hospice where they can manage his pain. We'll call and find out when there will be a place available.'

I felt like I was sleepwalking when I went back into the room to see Paul. Of course, I'd known it was coming; I just didn't think it would be so soon. I thought we might have had a few more weeks at least, if not months. I'd thought there would have been more of a gradual decline.

'Are you all right?' I asked him, and he said, 'Lindsey, I'm dying.' 'I know, darling, I know,' I said and he just stared at me. It was the first time I hadn't said 'You'll be all right.' I think he was relieved when I explained he was going to a hospice. He'd had enough. All he wanted was a good sleep. Patients have a sixth sense and I think he knew he'd reached rock bottom.

I helped him to have a shower that morning, placing a chair in the cubicle because he wasn't strong enough to stand up, and folding a towel over it so the bones of his bottom didn't hurt when he sat down. There was a full-length mirror in that bathroom and Paul screamed when he saw himself in it, with his ribs and his spine all sticking out.

'Lindsey, look at my body! It's awful.' He was horribly shocked. We didn't have a full-length mirror in the bathroom at home so it had been a while since he'd seen himself like this. He used to be so good-looking and so conscious of his looks that it was hard for him to see himself quite so ravaged by the cancer.

I said, 'Darling, you've lost a bit of weight but you're still gorgeous.' And all the while I was thinking, 'Jesus Christ, this is horrendous.'

It was the hardest thing I've ever had to do.

Anthony stayed with Paul at the Elland that night and the next morning, the Thursday, his pals Naeem and Stuart drove him over to the hospice in Huddersfield. I waited to give Alan a lift over and on the way I explained that he might be a bit shocked when he saw Paul in a wheelchair, and that he wasn't looking great. 'Just say "Hello, son!" as normal,' I asked. 'Don't let him see you're upset.'

When we got there, Paul had been put in a suite on his own, with a door leading out to some decking outside. It was lovely – like a nice, tasteful hotel bedroom with an ensuite bathroom rather than a hospital room. Paul was sitting outside in a yellow deckchair and seemed very cheery, although to my eyes he looked even worse than when I'd seen him the night before. Alan was devastated – I thought he was going to collapse but he managed to hold himself together. Just.

One of the first things they did when Paul got to the hospice was to put a device called a syringe driver into his arm. It's a tiny little box with a syringe in it and it was pumping morphine and other drugs into his arm at 20-minute intervals. As soon as it was working, Paul wasn't in pain any more and he seemed pretty cheerful, joking with the doctors and nurses.

One doctor asked, 'How are your waterworks?' and he was completely mystified when Paul said, 'If you pass go, you get £200' but I explained the joke – that we were playing Monopoly when I went into labour.

One nurse asked him where he wanted to be when it came to the 'final time'. Paul had always said he wanted to be at home, but this time he turned to me and said, 'What do you think, Linz? I quite like it here actually.' It was surreal to be having a casual conversation with your husband about where he was going to die. 'It's up to you, babes,' I said. 'Whatever you want.'

At that point, Paul was feeling so much better from the morphine that I'm convinced he didn't realize he was near the end. I think he thought he'd be home in a few days when he was rehydrated again.

I realized he didn't have long to go, though.

You just know.

*   *   *

This will sound odd to anyone who hasn't been in a similar situation, but over the last few weeks I was actually wishing for him to go. There was nothing left in his life any more. People ask how I can say such things, but I'm talking about a different Paul. I'm not talking about the Paul who was the centre of my world, who made me laugh and who loved me to bits. I'm not talking about a Paul who would have been around to see Evie grow up, who would have been the proud dad of more of our children. I'm not talking about a Paul who would have been the best snooker player in the world, who would have brought in so many more fans and achieved so much. I'm talking about a Paul who didn't know what day it was, who was riddled with cancer and crippled with pain. That was a Paul who wasn't himself, not the man I knew and not the man fans thought they knew. You wouldn't keep a dog in the pain he was in during his last month at home, and it would be cruel and wrong to try and keep someone in that state alive for another second because of what you wanted.

I do think that when he went into the hospice Paul just thought it was another bad patch. He thought there would be other options. He was always saying, 'Oh, there'll be something else to try, Linz; they're always coming up with new things.' I wouldn't shoot him down but I had accepted a couple of months before Paul died that the options had run out. There were people close to him who couldn't, or wouldn't face up to it – near the end, they were still saying that it was just a phase, that he was having a bad day. I did sometimes want to scream, 'Can't you see what's in front of you? Can't you see what's happening? He's wasting away, there's nothing left – he's not going to pull through, there isn't a miracle waiting to happen.'

Then there were those people who knew he was going to die but couldn't accept it was going to happen soon. I couldn't blame them: it was only a few weeks since the doctors had told us he'd have three to six months after they ran out of treatments to try, so in some ways it felt as though he was being cheated. Close friends and family like Nicky and some of the lads understood because they could see Paul, and they thought, 'We don't want you to be like that; we don't want you to be that ill because it's not you.'

Paul's parents held out as long as they possibly could. In fact, I think that until the day he went into the hospice they were still thinking, 'There's got to be something else.' But there wasn't. There isn't. It had to stop sometime. It took Alan and Kristina right until the last two days to accept that it was terminal. They thought their golden boy would hold on forever.

But when it's so close to the end, you can feel it.

Chapter Thirty-five

Letting go

5–9 October 2006

The day Paul went in to the hospice – Thursday 5 October – I knew it was the right decision. The people there were wonderful. They took all of the practical issues away from me and just left me and the family to be with Paul in his last hours. It was a huge relief, to be honest. Everything was comfortable there. The mattress on his bed was air-filled and moulded to his body to prevent bedsores. The room was light and sunny. The nurses were lovely. Above all, the most important thing was that they made sure he had no pain any more. I just wanted him to find peace.

On the Thursday afternoon, I had a very important chat with Paul – a chat about the future. He was joking with me, saying 'If I die, you're not allowed to go out with anyone else for at least a year.' I said, 'I don't want anyone else. No one could ever match up to you.'

'You'll meet someone else,' Paul predicted. 'You're young, you're gorgeous, of course you will. You'll get married and have kids with someone else.'

'If I have any other children, a brother or a sister for Evie, I'd want them to be yours, babes,' I told him. 'I'd like to use your sperm.'

'Would you really?' he asked, and seemed amazed but very pleased at the thought. 'Would you do that?'

The problem was that when he placed his samples in the sperm bank, we'd signed forms saying that it would require us both to consent if they were to be used in future. For me to be able to use that sperm after Paul passed away, we would have to change the consent form. Paul and I discussed it at length that afternoon and agreed that's what we wanted to do, but I had no idea how difficult it was going to be.

I called the department at St James' on Friday morning and explained to a woman on the phone what we wanted. 'No problem,' she said. 'You both have to come in here, see a counsellor and sign the form and then it will be legal.'

'I don't think you understand,' I said. 'Paul is in a hospice and he can't come in. Can't I just pick up the form and get him to sign it and then bring it back to you?'

'No, that wouldn't work, dear,' she said. 'He needs to chat to the counsellor to make sure he understands all the implications of what he's doing, so you'll have to get him to come here.'

I started crying down the phone, getting hysterical. 'We're running out of time,' I cried. 'You've got to help me.'

She rang off, saying she would see what she could do. I was beside myself, thinking it wasn't going to work out, that Evie would never have a brother or sister. The bureaucracy just seemed so idiotic. Surely we couldn't be the first couple to make a decision like this when one partner was on their deathbed?

Fortunately, common sense prevailed. That afternoon, two people from St James' came over to the hospice to chat to Paul. They explained all the procedures to him and he signed the forms and that was one problem out of the way at least.

We all took it in shifts to sit with Paul over that weekend. Me, his parents, his sister and her husband, Nicky, friends – all the people who loved him came to say goodbye. Everyone helped me to look after Evie so that I could spend as much time in the hospice as possible. I took her in briefly to see her daddy on the Friday, then Anthony brought her on Sunday morning, and Nicky brought her Monday lunchtime.

I telephoned Paul's closest friends and asked if they would like to see him one last time. Some of them were people who hadn't seen him for ages and had no idea how bad he was. One by one, I'd lead them up to his room, warning them not to look upset in front of him. Paul had brief but intimate con-versations with everyone; I think he knew he was saying goodbye because although they all left in pieces, each person said afterwards that he'd been very warm and funny and had something personal to say to them.

I called Darren Clarke and he came dashing over from Leicester but by the time he arrived on Saturday evening, Paul had started to go downhill. Daz had sworn he wouldn't cry but he couldn't believe how much Paul had deteriorated in the week since he'd last seen him: his eyes were closed and he just sat in the wheelchair mumbling that evening. Needless to say, Daz fell apart.

From then on, Paul didn't speak much any more but there were still the odd words, and grins, and he still kept trying to get up to do things for himself, as if he had no idea quite how ill he was.

Kris, a devout Catholic, sprinkled him with holy water at one point when she thought he was asleep. He opened his eyes and said, 'What tap did you get that from, Mum?'

On the Sunday evening, he decided he wanted to get to the toilet and he refused to be wheeled there in the wheelchair, so I put my arm round his shoulders and helped him to hobble painfully through. After he'd finished, he turned and fumbled to pull the flush. 'Don't worry about that, Paul,' I said, but he was insistent he was going to flush it. I couldn't believe he was still concerned about good manners at that stage. But it mattered to Paul.

On Sunday, 8 October, I had a chat with the doctors and they were concerned that he was still trying to get up and do things for himself that he really wasn't capable of. Following their advice, I agreed that they could sedate him a little more. I asked 'How long does he have?' and they didn't give a straight answer. They said it depended on how fast he deteriorated, but I knew by then things were changing by the hour.

I stayed over on Sunday night, dozing by the side of his bed in the same jeans and jumper. I wasn't sure how much he could understand any more, but during the night I whispered to Paul that I would make sure Evie knew everything about him. I told him that my life would go on for Evie's sake but it would never be the same without him in it. Nothing and nobody will ever be able to fill the big void in my life that he has left. I said everything I wanted to say, and most of all I told him how much I loved him.

Doctors and nurses came to check on him every so often. His body was still there, he was still breathing, but I knew my Paul was never coming back. He'd never look at me again or kiss me or hold me or make me laugh. My throat was aching and my eyes stinging from not letting myself cry. If he did come round, I didn't want him to see me upset. He'd always taken his lead from me and I didn't want to let him know just how unbearable this was.

In the early hours of the morning, one doctor said to me that he'd have expected Paul to have gone by now. It was as if he was still fighting away, not giving up. From time to time he groaned, even though he was so heavily sedated.

What was he holding on for?

It was then a thought occurred to me. Paul had relied on me so much to tell him what to do since he was first diagnosed, that he wouldn't do a thing without seeing how I was going to approach it.

He was waiting.

He was waiting for me to tell him it was all right to die.

There was a split second when I thought I couldn't do it. I just couldn't do it, but then something welled up inside of me and I felt a strength greater than anything I'd felt for months. Of course I could.

'Look, babes, you've been fighting for a long time,' I whispered. My voice jumped, my throat felt as if it was closing. 'But it's OK. You can go now. You can stop fighting.'

He sighed in his sleep. I had no way of telling whether he had heard or not.

All day Monday, his mum, Leanne and I sat by his bed, with different family members coming and going. I remember we watched *West Side Story* on video. I massaged Paul's legs and feet, because they had become very swollen. We brushed his hair, brushed his teeth, told stories and chatted – not about anything important, just general chit-chat.

About seven o'clock *Emmerdale* came on the telly and a nurse came in and asked if we would all like to go and have a cup of tea while she changed Paul's bed. Joanne and I were the first back in the room after they'd finished and we saw straight away that Paul was in a different position and his breathing was so shallow that his chest didn't seem to be moving at all. Joanne ran to find the rest of the family and told them to get there – fast. His mum, dad, Leanne and her husband Adam, his cousins Craig and Joanne, and his Auntie Teresa all came rushing in. I sat on the bed and held his right hand. Kris held his left hand.

It was as if Paul was waiting for us all to get there. As soon as we were all huddled round the bed, he took one last, deep breath and then he left us.

Chapter Thirty-six

Goodbye, my love

*P*aul died at five to eight on the evening of Monday 9 October 2006. It was five days before his twenty-eighth birthday.

I could tell straight away that he'd gone.

'I love you, babes,' I whispered in his ear.

Alan was so calm. 'You'll be all right, Paul,' he said. 'My dad will find you in Heaven – he'll look after you.'

No one cried. There was this spooky calm and everyone was talking, saying the most lovely things. I didn't want to let go of his hand but everyone else wanted to touch him, to kiss him, and there wasn't enough of him to go round. We all felt filled with the most incredible feeling of love.

A nurse came in to shut his eyes but she couldn't get the lids to go all the way down. Paul had always slept with his eyes slightly open – 'To keep an eye on you,' he'd joke to me. Evie does the same thing.

I unfastened the dogtag necklace, which I had bought for him as a wedding present, then I removed his diamond stud earring. I'd been wearing the other one of the pair since the day he went into the hospice. I also put on that white dressing gown he'd been wearing for the last few months, because it still smelled of him.

After about 10 minutes, we noticed Paul's hand was getting cold and we pulled up the covers to warm him, knowing all the while it was crazy. At least we could hug him now without hurting him. His face looked so peaceful and handsome, no longer twisted with pain. There was even what looked like a little half smile on his lips. I felt numb at that stage. I think when someone you love dies, you feel anaesthetized for the first little while and it's weeks later that you begin to experience the loss properly.

Alan and Kris said they would stay the night with Paul – they didn't want to leave their son on his own, and I understood that, but I needed to get home. I rang my parents and was astonished when my big, strong father burst into tears on the phone. I rang my sister. I rang Nicky and she said she'd come straight over because she wanted to say goodbye to Paul. I rang Brandon, and he was in the departure lounge at an airport in Barbados, waiting for a flight home. Naeem had called him the day before to say the end was near and he'd got on the first flight he could but too late to see Paul again. He cried in that airport for a full two hours.

News of Paul's death got out to the media quickly and a reporter rang the hospice at 9pm wanting me to comment; I just told the nurse they could get lost. Nicky arrived soon after that to say goodbye to her baby cousin and to look after me.

'Why don't you come back and stay at ours, Linz?' she

asked, hugging me, but I knew I wanted to be in my own house. She said she would come to mine, then – that I should-n't be on my own.

I kissed Paul one last time and said 'Love you!' then I drove Nicky and myself back home. I just felt so numb and distant from everything. It all seemed so unreal. We sat in my sitting room with a cup of tea and both took one of Paul's sleeping tablets. We didn't talk much but just sat in silence. Occasionally Nicky would say, 'Are you OK, babes?' and I'd nod automatically.

We cuddled up together in our bed and I slept soundly for the first time in months. Evie was staying at my mum and dad's, and the sound of Paul moaning and groaning in his sleep beside me was no longer there.

When I woke the next morning, there were lots of jobs to be getting on with – including dealing with the pack of photog-raphers and journalists who were camped at the end of our drive. I gave a press statement, saying that I didn't want to mourn but I wanted to celebrate Paul's life.

The next few days are blurry even now.

Brandon got back, and he and I and Paul's parents met with the funeral directors. I told them that I wanted Paul to be dressed in his snooker outfit, including his dickie bow, waistcoat and white shirt. I ironed all his clothes before handing them over. He always felt cold during the cancer treatments, so I gave them some thermal socks to put on his feet to keep them warm. He loved his thermals. I knew it was daft but I still did it. That's the strange thing – you go from one extreme to the other. One minute you're being really practical and sensible, and the next you're wanting thermal socks put on your husband's lifeless body. Of course I knew it wasn't real, I wasn't thinking it would help; but you're so desperate to do something that sometimes you grasp at things that are mad.

I just wanted to be able to look after him again.

I loved looking after him.

The morning after Paul died, I couldn't get the image out of my head of his face just after he died. It was peaceful, he wasn't in pain, but it wasn't my Paul, the guy who had more life in him than anyone I'd ever met. Gradually, over the next two days, this image was replaced with a picture of him looking gorgeous, with his long hair – before he started chemo, before he had it cut. It was such a nice image that when they asked me on the Wednesday if I wanted to see Paul's body in the Chapel of Rest, I said no. I wanted to remember him healthy and strong and cheeky and gorgeous. Kris is very religious, so she went every day right up until they had to close the coffin, and she said he looked lovely, very peaceful.

A faith healer brought me a crucifix to place in Paul's right hand, with a note saying: 'It is from a place called Medjugorje in Bosnia-Herzegovina, a very special place where Our Lady appears. It is a place of calm and peace.' I gave it to the undertaker who promised to make sure it was done before the cremation.

It was Paul's birthday on the Saturday, so I asked them to

put his birthday cards and some photos of him and Evie together in the coffin as well.

The thanksgiving and funeral was held at Leeds Parish Church on Thursday 19 October 2006 at 2pm. It had taken us 10 days to make all the preparations because we had been warned that the turnout was going to be huge and it was important that all the arrangements worked smoothly. Paul's closed coffin stood in the church for two days before the service, along with a book of condolence in which people could write messages, and there were some beautiful ones that gave me a lot of comfort. There were thousands of messages in there, each one of them heartfelt and lovely.

Brandon and I put a lot of thought into the booklet announcing the order of service. The front showed two beautiful pictures of Paul. On the left-hand side he was in his snooker uniform: black trousers, black waistcoat and black bow tie with a crisp, white shirt. The very clothes we cremated him in. He was holding a snooker cue in his hand and his hair was quite long, past chin length. He wasn't smiling, but it was still my Paul. On the right-hand side of the front cover was another picture in which his hair was more dishevelled and he was wearing a patterned shirt, open to show a white t-shirt, casual trousers and a loose scarf. He stood with his hands in his pockets, again with a serious look on his face, but gorgeous. The photographs had been blended together so that you couldn't see a line between them – you were just looking at two images, the two sides of Paul Hunter. He looked so well, so healthy – but underneath were the words that told the rest of the story:

A Thanksgiving for the Life of Paul Alan Hunter

And then, on the back cover, as if there could be any doubt, were his name and the dates of his birth and death.

Paul Alan Hunter
1978–2006

So stark, so unforgiving. The photograph on the back was a black and white one. Paul wasn't looking at the camera – he was in his snooker uniform again and looking up to the right. He looked poignant. He looked thoughtful. He looked like he hadn't looked for so very long.

Inside the booklet, there was a page of four photos show-ing Paul playing snooker and winning. He looked so perfect, golden and happy. Another shot shows him sitting in the sunshine, in jeans and a black top. Then, at the end, there is a picture of the three of us. Our family. Paul holding Evie and kissing the side of her head. Evie in the middle of us staring at the camera with her huge blue eyes, while I look at Paul from the other side. Just normal people having to cope with extraordinary things.

All of the pictures were chosen with great care in the week leading up to the funeral. I love those pictures and I know that they touched a lot of people, because Paul just looks absolutely awesome in them. Each one of them means something to me and, I'm sure, to the many other people who loved and knew Paul. It was hard, though, to look at a 16-page booklet that basically confirmed what my heart knew all too well – my husband was dead.

The order of service began by welcoming everyone to the church and acknowledging that everyone there would have their very own special memories of Paul. Lots of the words could apply to anyone who had died too soon, but there were also plenty of clues about how Paul had affected people and how he meant so much to so many. And not everyone has instructions in their funeral order of service about how to behave when the Lord Mayor and other dignitaries arrive.

The day of the funeral came and I had a huge lump in my throat from the moment I got up, but I knew I just had to get through it. I'd decided that Evie should be there too, even though she wouldn't know what was going on as she was still only 10 months old. It helped me to be able to cling to her at the saddest moments, and I suppose it underlined for everyone there just how much Paul had lost. He'd lost the chance to see his daughter growing up, to hear her first proper words and watch her first steps, and so much else.

We'd chosen the flowers with great care. On the hearse, the words 'My Daddy' were spelled out in pink orchids, and next to a photograph of Paul there was a card that said 'From your princess'. Other floral tributes said 'Son' and 'Bro' and 'Legend'. I followed, feeling completely sick and unreal. Six pallbearers – Matthew Stevens, Darren Clarke, Jimmie Michie, Darren Shaw, Naeem and Bear, all of Paul's closest snooker friends – carried the coffin into the church.

In fact, the snooker world was out in force that day – Steve Davis, Ronnie O'Sullivan, Jimmy White, Joe Johnson, John Parrott, Willie Thorne, Dennis Taylor and John Virgo were among the champions past and present who came to pay their respects. As we walked in we went through this tunnel of professional snooker players – dozens and dozens of them. The church was full to bursting and hundreds of snooker fans stood outside, many of them unable to hold back the tears.

The opening music was 'Going to Fly Now' from *Rocky III*. It was the music that Paul often played in his dressing room before matches to gear himself up – and I play it to this day when I need to get myself ready for something. After that, there was a welcome by the Minister which included the words:

We have come before God today to remember Paul Hunter; to give thanks for his life; to commend him to God his merciful redeemer and judge; to commit his body to be cremated, and to comfort one another in our grief; in the hope that is ours through the death and resurrection of Jesus Christ.

Paul wasn't religious and neither was I – but as I heard the sobs and intakes of breath around me, I realized that these words would comfort some. I just focused throughout on the one thing I knew to be true – that wasn't Paul in the box. My Paul, the Paul I knew and loved, had gone. When his body gave up, when he finally closed his eyes and went to sleep, he was free of the pain that he had borne so bravely for months on end. I couldn't weep, I couldn't scream with loss for him – because I was glad that he had been spared any more agony.

After the welcome, we all sang 'Praise my soul, the King of Heaven', before the Prayers of Penitence. Then came perhaps the hardest part: the three personal tributes to Paul. Firstly, Alan said a few words.

> *Seeing family, friends, and friends from the snooker world, our world, would make our son Paul so proud knowing that so many loved him. He would say, 'I'm glad there's a good turnout.' It shows to Paul's mum, myself, Leanne, Lindsey and Evie Rose and all the family just how much our beautiful son was loved. Paul and Lindsey were so happy, and when Evie Rose came along, Paul came into his own as a great father. We all shared a laugh and a drink with Paul, we all know Paul loved the fast lane – but that's not why we are here today. Paul said to me, not long ago, 'I've just been dealt a bad card.' He never once said, 'Why me?' He was so strong to the very end, for all the family. We will miss you so much. We are all so proud of you, Paul.*

We all listened as Psalm 121 was sung by the choir, then Paul's cousin Anthony gave a speech. He said:

> *Thank you again for coming; it means so much to all of us. I've known Paul all his life; we were very close cousins and best friends. Paul will always be Paul to me and the rest of his family. We treasured so many great memories together and we were there for each other. I'm so proud that I was*

there for him when he needed me most. Deep down I never gave up hope and tried to stay as positive as I could in a horrible situation. We did talk about what could happen, and he would say: 'Whatever will be, will be.' We all thought the world of Paul, for who he is, and for what he has achieved. We didn't realize just how many hearts he touched, not just with his family and friends, but people from all around the world. I don't think he realized that either, which goes to show what a unique, charismatic, modest guy he was. He was a fighter, through and through. We saw that on and off the table. He never gave up; right to the very end he battled against the cancer. As much as I waffled on and made the simplest things complicated, I hope that I played a part in keeping his spirit alive.

Anthony read out the words from a song they'd both liked as kids:

*Fight till you drop, never stop
Can't give up until you reach the top.*

He admitted that when it finished, they'd always leap up and practise some karate moves on each other in the middle of the living room, and continued:

I never did tell Auntie I broke her expensive ornament; I blamed it on Paul! Paul had time for everybody, something that we as his family, friends and followers should have too. I'll always remember on his eighteenth birthday I interviewed

*him for an assignment at college. It took us 35 takes because
we were laughing so much it hurt and it was hard to
concentrate. That's the Paul I know, that's the Paul we all
know, always with a smile on his face, that cheeky grin, the
answer he had for everything, and the odd double vodka.
Paul gave us so much, he gave us himself, his magnetic
personality, his generosity, his looks, his hairstyles, and above
all his courage and determination. I'm glad you're at peace
now, Paul, and we'll love you always and forever.*

Anthony's words were followed by a Gaelic blessing sung
by the choir and then Sir Rodney Walker of the World
Snooker Association gave a tribute. There was a reading
(John 14:1–6) before a further hymn and the Address by the
Rector of Leeds, Reverend Canon Tony Bundock.

There were more hymns and then it was my turn. My stomach was in knots but I had said I would read a poem written by
Don Clarke, the father of Paul's friend Darren, who had been
such a support to us – and I was determined to get through it
without breaking down and making a fool of myself. In fact,
when I stood up at the podium, I felt a calm strength fill me. I
looked out at the sea of faces and read it as expressively as I
could, because I agreed with every single word.

A Tribute to a Champion

*There's one bright star in the heavens tonight and oh how it
    shines for all to see,
for this star is special, for it has a smile and laughter for now
    it is free.*

Free from all pain and sorrow, its battle for life has ended,
for it has now a new tomorrow and its body is now fully
*   mended.*

But it's not just a star in the heavens, where it shines so
*   brightly and proud,*
for this star on earth was a champion, and oh how it thrilled
*   all the crowd.*

Now this star was blessed with talent, that only the best are
*   allowed,*
so be grateful if you ever met him, and if you were his friend,
*   then be proud.*

He played the game that he loved, he played with a passion so
*   rare,*
and all of the crowds that saw him were privileged because
*   they were there.*

So, if you stood at the great gates of heaven, with one look
*   then you would understand,*
for amongst a great host of angels, would be one with a cue
*   in his hand.*

Safe with the Lord now, Paul. God bless.

As I sat down, I could hear weeping all around me. I had
done my bit, though. I got through it for Paul.

As the service ended, music began. This time, it was

'Amazed' – the song we had played at our wedding; the song that reminded us both constantly of how amazed we really were by each other.

At the funeral, everyone said that Paul was one of snooker's brightest stars and could easily have gone on to be a world champion. Willie Thorne related that Paul always told him he didn't mind the chemotherapy making his hair drop out as long as he didn't end up looking like Willie Thorne! He said that the number of players who had turned up that day showed just what the world thought about Paul.

In interviews for the media, Willie said: 'I admired the kid so much; he battled so very hard.' Dennis Taylor said: 'It's a dreadfully sad loss. He would have been the World Champion, that's for sure.' Alex 'Hurricane' Higgins agreed: 'Paul could have become World Champ. He was a great bloke and a great snooker player.'

To me, it was all so much simpler than that.

He was just my Paul.

Chapter Thirty-seven

Paul's legacy

October–December 2006

In the weeks after the funeral, I kept myself as busy as possible, looking after Evie, going back to work, and dealing with practical matters – anything to distract myself from the reality of what had just happened. Of course, there were moments when I curled up in a ball and cried bitter, painful tears for everything that Evie, Paul and I had lost, for the family we could have been. But it would be an insult to Paul if I dwelled on the negative. I'm alive and he's not. He'd do anything to be here right now but it just wasn't possible, so I've got to make the best of it for his sake. That's what he'd tell me to do if he could: 'Get your arse in gear, Linz,' he'd say, and quite right too.

There are certain little things – daft things maybe – that I do. I've worn his diamond earrings ever since he died. I wear his boxer shorts in bed – partly because they're comfy – and for the first few months I always slept on his side of the bed. I also wear some of his zippy tops and t-shirts but not necessarily for sentimental reasons; lots of girls wear their partners' clothes when they want to slouch around at home. The only difference is that Paul is not here when I do it. Kris has got some of his clothes as well, and I gave his snooker cue to Alan, because I know that's what Paul would have wanted.

There were so many letters and cards of condolence that, even to this day, I am staggered. We had received over five hundred cards and letters in the days after it was first announced that Paul had cancer – and I have them all even now – but, after his death, it was phenomenal. Some of the letters appear in an appendix at the end of this book so I can share some of the beautiful sentiments they expressed. I knew that Paul was liked, loved even, by many people he'd encountered over the years, but I was still enormously heartened at how many of them took the time to contact me and share their feelings.

I hadn't given any thought as yet to what we would do with Paul's ashes. Kris and Alan had taken them home after the cremation and kept them beside a photo of Evie. I was torn between trying to be really practical and thinking, That's not Paul, that's just a box of ashes, and a strange emotional feeling – That's all I've got left, that's all there is of him.

One morning in November I woke up and thought, I wonder if Paul can see me? If he can, is he wondering why I haven't got his ashes? Does he think that I don't care? I didn't want him to think I wasn't bothered, so I asked Alan and Kris if they would mind if I took the ashes, and they agreed. When I brought the box home, I kept it in the kitchen to begin with. Looking at it took my breath away – it was made of exactly the same wood as Paul's coffin and had the exact same plaque with his name and dates of birth and death on it. I felt winded at first looking at it.

I kept the box in the kitchen for a bit, then I put him in the snooker room because he loved it so much in there. I surrounded the box with bottles of champagne and vodka because he'd had some great times in that room and it had been full of wonderful memories; in a funny way, I wanted to give him a bit of that back.

Our first Christmas without Paul came quickly – the two months just flew by and I knew that I had to have things planned. In some ways, I was glad that he'd died before Christmas so that we didn't spend 25 December by his bedside in a hospital or hospice, watching him in pain, knowing that this would be his last Christmas. As it was, I had a plan; I knew what Evie and I were going to do.

One day when he was in the hospice, Paul had woken up and said to me out of the blue: 'Can we have a tree in the bedroom so that it really feels like Christmas this year?' He was like a little boy, so hyped up on it. 'Of course we can, babes!' I told him, despite being pretty sure that he wouldn't see 25 December. So as Christmas approached, I put up a tree in our bedroom. Paul loved the feeling of Christmas, loved the excitement, and I tended to put up a couple of trees anyway. He always had a childlike quality and he could always make you feel the same excitement he was feeling. So, the first year without him, I decided we would have a proper Christmas, just as we would have done if he had been there, if he had been well. I hope he still felt it; I hope he was still excited.

I brought his ashes back into the kitchen and placed them on a table, surrounded by pictures of Evie and her little advent calendar. I spoke to that box every day, and told people 'Paul's in the kitchen!' They probably thought I was mad, but I didn't care.

Everyone wanted us to stay over at their houses on Christmas Eve but I wanted to do what I always do. There are some things that you don't want to change – or change too quickly. I needed some continuity. Paul and I used to 'do the rounds' on Christmas Eve, dropping off presents for everyone, and I did that as usual, then came back to our house to spend the night.

On Christmas morning, I couldn't help myself thinking back to the previous year, which had been so wonderful – I was in labour, our baby was coming, and we were together. But I had to stop myself dwelling on that sort of thing – I had to keep going. When I went to my parents' house and then Paul's parents' house that day, I took the casket with me. I didn't want him to miss out on any of the fun.

For Evie's first birthday, on Boxing Day, I'd decided to throw a party. At first, I thought I'd just invite friends with children, but then I realized that other friends would find Evie's first birthday hard too because they would be thinking about how proud Paul would have been and how much he was missing. There were also some people that I hadn't seen for a while, as it had all been so hectic since Paul's death. So, in the end, I invited about 17 kids each with their parents, and then about 20 other friends who didn't have kids.

On Evie's birthday morning, she slept in until about half

past nine, which was the latest she'd ever managed. The little soul must have been worn out from all the excitement of the day before, or maybe her Daddy's sleeping gene was kicking in!

When she woke, I dressed her in a brand new outfit and got to work preparing the house. It all looked lovely and, by keeping myself so busy, I didn't have time to stop and think about the one thing that was missing. Paul.

Everybody arrived at about one o'clock and, within minutes, it was bedlam. I had put '1pm–5pm' on the invitations on purpose, because this was just a party for Evie. I didn't want everyone to think this was another of the parties Paul and I used to have, when no one would get home until the next day. At this party, I didn't want anyone to drink too much because then they would get depressed – and this was meant to be Evie's day, not a wake.

Evie was awake at one o'clock when they all arrived, but she only lasted about an hour after that, poor thing. The house was absolutely stuffed with people and I kept thinking that, not only could I not dwell on Paul's absence, but I had to stop others from doing the same thing. I had to keep everybody up, up, up. I don't doubt for a second that it was hard for friends and family. That was the house I'd lived in with Paul and now he was gone. Some of them, lots of them, hadn't been there since well before Paul had died. Several people said that going into the games room was especially hard because they expected him to be standing behind the bar. That was where the biggest gap was; to be honest, he wouldn't have been sitting quietly with Evie on his lap – he'd have been getting everyone else a drink behind the optics. He would probably have been carrying her around and I know he would have been bursting with pride. His little angel, one year old.

Paul's friend Bear took his place behind the bar serving drinks, people were playing pool and it looked like a normal party on the surface, but it was so different from all the wild ones we'd had there. I had deliberately not bought too much booze, because I didn't want things to get maudlin. I remember a party we'd had one year when we bought six bottles of vodka, two bottles of brandy and everything else we could think of, and we told people to bring what they wanted as well. Everything got drunk – there wasn't a drop left. Now, I had 15 kids on the floor in the lounge watching *Harry Potter* and eating snacks, while I tried to get a game of pass-the-parcel going amongst the younger ones.

Everyone was trying to take as many photos of Evie and the house as possible because I had warned them that I planned to move after the New Year, as soon as I could get things organized. It reminded me of the months when I was constantly taking pictures of Paul and Evie together, because I was so scared of losing out on memories for her future. I could see people taking all these pictures of Evie and nearly crying while they were doing it, and I knew they were all thinking, Paul should be here. I wanted to tell them, 'No, he shouldn't!' because it would have been awful. I know everyone deals with the pain of a loss differently but you can't keep someone hanging on in agony and despair just because you want them to be there for a certain date on the calendar.

I think a lot of people don't understand me; since Paul was diagnosed, and certainly since he died, I haven't always acted in the way the rest of the world expects me to act. If I had been sobbing or wailing that *my* husband couldn't be there for *my* baby daughter's first birthday then perhaps they would have found this easier to relate to. At least then I'd be acting the conventional widow's role and they could hug me and pat me on the back and cry along with me. Well, I'm not like that and I loved Paul too much to pray for him to hang on when he was in such intolerable pain.

Anyway, it was a nice party, a really nice day, but I'd never do it again – I don't care what it takes, I'll find another location to have a party for her on Boxing Day every year from now on. That way, I'll make sure the memories are about Evie's future, not her past. That's what Paul would have wanted for his daughter too.

Chapter Thirty-eight

Life goes on

People always ask how I've coped. I think it's just in me to be like this. I suppose I've changed a bit over the years – everyone does. Even with little things, practical things. Our Tracy loves to cook but, like my mum, I was never that bothered. However, once I was settled in Batley with Paul, I got better at it, partly because it made him happy if I made him nice meals, but also just as part of growing up.

You can't plan for things like this – God help anyone who goes into their marriage knowing that their husband is going to die in a couple of years – but if you've got the foundations anyway, you stand a much better chance. If I'd had different parents, a different upbringing, maybe I would have crumbled.

I still keep things behind different doors in my mind so that I don't have to deal with them all at once. It's one of the ways that I manage to stay positive and look to the future, rather than dwelling on what has gone. I can take them out and look at them one by one, and that way it stays manageable. Just.

*   *   *

One of the biggest things for me to make a decision about was the house in Batley. That was our house – but there wasn't going to be an 'us' any more. It had fantastic memories – Paul's face when we moved in, all the parties, bringing Evie home from hospital. Obviously there were dark times too. During the last two years in the house in Batley, Paul had been poorly. There was so much pain and illness locked up in it. In the last weeks of his life, I got it into my head that I didn't want to stay there when he'd gone. If Paul had still been here, it would have been our home forever. We'd be trying for another baby by now, I guess.

But the thing that really made up my mind to move was the thought that every time a friend came round, they'd always remember Paul. They would have memories of him being ill there that would probably overwhelm the good memories. They would always feel that he was missing. It would turn into a house full of sadness and I could not have Evie brought up in that sort of environment. She will know everything about her daddy, and I will burst with pride each time I tell her something new, but I didn't want people always pointing out things to her and saying what Paul was like in that house. I was so determined just to preserve the good memories.

Tracy and Chris had got into property developing and they'd built a new house next to their existing one. However, they actually ended up staying there for a while, and any time Paul visited he loved it to pieces. He'd say, 'I love these doors, Linz; I love this room,' and go on and on. In fact, he loved everything that Tracy and Chris did to it; he really liked their taste. I remember one night going round and him saying to me, 'Linz, their nibbles are better than ours! Can we have them in little bowls like this?' It wasn't envy – he just admired them and looked up to them.

Tracy and Chris moved back to the original house after a bit and decided to put the other one up for sale just as I was putting our Batley house on the market. It all fell into place as we were chatting one day. 'Lindsey,' said Tracy, 'buy this. Buy this house! We'll be next to each other all the time. Evie can play with Matthew and Eloise whenever she wants, and you'll have family yards away to help you out if you need it.' She was right. It was ideal. I know my mum and dad think that it's lovely, us living next door to each other, and I agree. The three little cousins see each other constantly. We don't have to plan visits because they just run in and out of each other's houses all the time. Evie copies everything Matthew and Eloise do, and they treat her like a little sister.

Mum says she is glad that I could move on; she didn't want me stuck in Batley on my own thinking I had to stay there because of Paul's memory. Dad said, 'It's marvellous you and Tracy live next to each other; it'll give you the opportunity to go to the next stage in your life with Tracy by your side. You'll always love Paul but you've made the decision to move on with your life, and that's the right thing to do.'

There were some practical things to be done, and some of these nearly pushed me over the edge. Selling Paul's beloved BMW was hard, so hard. He loved his car so much. I couldn't bear being at home to watch as it was driven away for the last time.

I always slept on his side of the bed before we moved house. After I moved into my new place and got a new bed, I tended to sleep in the middle of the bed – not exactly on Paul's side, but closer to it than I did before he died.

I'm getting through step by step. It's by no means easy, and often the tears are never far away, but tiny bits of normality do start to seep back, bit by bit. And Evie needs me. She is my light and reminds me that Paul's love is always around me. I think I'm doing quite well on the whole.

For Kris and Alan, it has been tougher. To lose your own child is horrendous. Because they found it so hard to accept how ill Paul was, and they didn't believe he was dying right up until the end, it came as much more of a shock when it happened. They had to get over the shock of his death before they could even start grieving. To this day, their house is like a shrine, with his photographs on every wall and some of his trophies on display.

When you lose your husband and the father of your child, you just have to get through things day by day. I know it's the same for Alan and Kris, trying to come to terms with the loss of their wonderful son.

I miss him. We all do.

I miss holding Paul's hand. I miss sharing the nice, emotional times. You can have a physical relationship with anyone, but you can't share your life with just anyone. I want him to cuddle me again.

What is hard to accept is never having any new photos,

any new memories of him, ever again. I know that when Kris sees photographs of him that she doesn't have, she immediately makes a copy and I can understand that. For her, perhaps it's like getting a new memory – like managing to get a bit of her son's life that she didn't have before. At a time when you can never ever get any new memories from the future, maybe you should get as much of the past as you can.

Sundays are the hardest. That's the day when everybody does family things. Paul had wanted to have a baby for so long. Before Evie was born, he used to say that he would never be able to change a nappy in front of anyone in case he made a mess of it, yet he got the hang of it so quickly and even when he was feeling awful, he'd do what he could. He'd be so proud pushing the buggy with his daughter in it. He'd have loved the little things – taking her to the park, reading her bedtime stories. There would have been times when his two worlds would have collided. Paul Hunter the dad would have been Paul Hunter the snooker champion at the same time. I can just imagine him walking round the Crucible talking to fans and other players with little Evie in his arms.

And some of that has happened.

One of the biggest moments after Paul's death was at the BBC Sports Personality of the Year awards on 10 December 2006. At every ceremony, there is an award in the name of Helen Rollason, one of their presenters who died of cancer. Barely months after his death, I was contacted by the BBC to say that they wanted Paul to receive Helen's award for bravery posthumously. This was going to be the first time that the BBC had broadcast the programme live from out-side the studios, and it was going to be a huge event in front of 10,000 people in the arena, and millions on television.

The BBC put together a film reflecting on Paul's life and achievements, and they were also going to go live to a snooker match where some of the big names playing that day would broadcast their tributes to Paul. After that, they'd ask me to accept the award. Would I do it? Would I stand in front of millions watching a film of my dead husband; a film designed to make people cry at what had been lost?

I didn't take a second to make my decision.

Of course I would.

What's more, I wanted to make a speech too. This was for Paul.

On the night, Brandon took me aside and said, 'Lindsey, I know what's coming up. I've seen the film and it's heart-breaking. There are players talking about Paul and it's just awful to see how much he meant to everyone and how much he's missed. Don't watch it because you'll be so upset.'

I didn't feel like that. I wanted to see it. I told Brandon, 'When I see Paul, it makes me stronger. I'm doing this for him. I won't let him down.'

Brandon walked off and I know he was in tears when they showed it. I composed myself as I stood there watching it. I knew what I had to do.

In the film, his fellow snooker players said that Paul was such a character and brought something completely differ-ent to the game. They said that they always wondered whether he'd be wearing something new when he came out, like the bandanna – he was one of those people who could get away with anything. Lots of them commented on the fact that Paul was very gracious, and if you didn't look at the score line you'd never actually know whether he was down and losing, or racing ahead. I was in the film too. They'd interviewed me and all I could really say was: 'We've got Evie Rose with us here now, and she's such a tribute to Paul.' It ends with Ronnie saying that Paul Hunter had 27 years of happiness.

Then Gary Lineker asked the crowd to welcome me.

The camera panned across the audience and there were so many people in floods of tears. Jimmy White was standing next to Gary waiting for me, and it looked as if he was going to break down any second. There was a deafening burst of applause as they played some opera music and I walked out to see all these people who had truly loved my husband. I knew that people were holding their breath to see if I would get overcome with emotion – but I knew what I had to say:

> *It's hard to find the words to describe a man like Paul Hunter – he didn't have a pretentious bone in his body. In the challenging arena of snooker, he always felt privileged to be in the same room as others. In defeat he was a true sportsman. His life may have been cut short but the people who were close to him feel lucky to have known him. I was lucky enough to fall in love with the man of my dreams. He has left me our daughter, Evie Rose. She really is the double of her father. I will be proud to tell her: your daddy was Paul Hunter.*

It was a strange feeling. Everyone there was thinking about Paul at the same moment. Paul's picture was behind me, people were in tears, lots of his friends were feeling the loss – but I was calm. I was paying proud tribute to my own husband and there was no way I was going to fail him.

Zara Phillips had won the Sports Personality of the Year award, so she gave a speech too. One day after Paul died I had got home to find some gorgeous flowers and a card from her saying, 'Thinking of you, love Zara.' Paul had met her a couple of times through sporting functions, so it was very nice of her to do that. At the awards, I went over to her early in the evening and said, 'Thanks for the flowers,' and she just said she was glad I had got them.

I didn't see her again until the end of the ceremony when I went over to say congratulations – hers was the last and main award of the night. I told her she deserved it, and she said, laughing, 'You cow! It's not really my night after you get up there and make that amazing speech. It was fantastic – and I can't even say a bloody thing apart from "amazing" over and over again! We're taught how to do public speaking for years and you did so much better than me!'

She was lovely that evening, and it just goes to show yet again that there were no barriers between Paul and other sportspeople; they all mixed together and they all liked him, every single one.

His memory was so strong.

*   *   *

Whenever something like that happens – especially when I laugh about something that Paul has played a part in – the loss hits me. I wrote on his funeral bouquet 'Paul, you are and always will be the only one. You have my heart.'

He does.

He always did.

He always will.

And what he gave me was so much more than a scrapbook full of clippings.

He gave me the faith in myself to keep going.

I can't even begin to say how much I miss him – but the love we built together was so strong that it will live on forever. I have to keep saying the same thing – thanks Paul, thanks for everything. I'll hold your love in my heart for as long as I live.

In the final battle, your spirit proved stronger than anyone could ever have imagined.

You showed them all.

You were unbreakable.

Epilogue

Dear Paul –

There is so much I want to say to you, so much I want to tell you. Someone once asked me what I would do if I could have one last hour with you (she said I had to keep it clean!).

I know what my first choice would be. I'd put Evie in the room with you and walk out – I so want you to have time with her, to have time together.

If I did have to use the time for me, I'd want to share everything about our beautiful baby girl with you. My family and friends have been wonderful, and they share in my joy every time Evie reaches another milestone.

But they aren't you.
They aren't her daddy.

I want to tell you about her personality. She's so like you, Paul! She loves to show off, to make people laugh, to be an entertainer. You were like that, as we all know – maybe it's in her blood. The faces she pulls are faces that you pulled. She saw you for so little time that she can't really have picked anything up from you, and yet she almost looks as if she's copying what you used to do at times.

I want you to see her.
I want you to see her so much.

I know that if you were here, you'd be winding me up good and proper. You'd be saying that she's all you, that she's her daddy's girl, and you'd be chuffed to bits about it. I wouldn't mind because what would be better than for that to be really happening? We'd be trying for a baby brother or sister for Evie round about now. I'll have to make that decision at some point, and you might be a daddy again without ever knowing it. This isn't the time to settle such a thing, it's too soon, but I wish you were here to discuss it with me.

I don't think I'd need to talk about myself, because I think you'd know what I've been doing since you died. You'd know that I've kept on with things, that I've tried my absolute best to do the right things for us. I know that you wouldn't want me to focus on bad stuff, and I wouldn't waste a precious second with you by dwelling on anything negative.

I would want to try and make you understand just how many people cared for you and what an impact you made in your 27 years.

Unbreakable

I want to thank you for the happiness and love you gave me and for the whole feeling we had together of being complete.

I want to thank you for Evie.
For the life you've left us with.
For the friends you gave me.
For the memories of the years together.
For the things that are still happening because of you.

I'd still pick you, Paul.

Even if I knew we had to go through it all again, I'd still pick you, babes. I'd still pick you.

Your wife, Lindsey xxx

Letters for Paul

Amongst the hundreds of letters I received after Paul died were some from his sponsors and most told of how they had ended up closer to Paul than they would ever have thought in a 'professional' relationship:

My dear Lindsey
There are no words that could possibly express adequately how
everyone at Cantor feels about their personal and collective loss –
your beloved Paul. To say that we are absolutely devastated is a
supreme understatement. The last two years must have been living
hell. Paul seemed to bear his illness stoically and with great
fortitude. But after all, through his quietly spoken demeanour, he
was always a hugely competitive and talented person, so it is
ridiculous to have expected any other approach to the massive task
in hand. Paul was a marvellous ambassador for our company.
All of us will remember his impish smile, his great charm, his
kindness and his cheeky-chappy personality. You and your family
are constantly in our thoughts. Twenty-seven is no age at all. It is

the injustice that is so hard for everyone to cope with. Hopefully the love and affection you will receive from your family and host of friends will help to sustain you in your terrible loss.

Yours sincerely, David Buik, Cantor Fitzgerald

Dear Lindsey

It has taken me a week to be able to put pen to paper to write to you. It was only after I heard the news about Paul that I realized quite how fond of him I had become. I have said to so many people that the sponsor-player relationship with Paul quickly became a friendship. It was impossible not to become a friend of Paul's – he was so normal, just a really decent human being. I have never met such a humble man in my life – he had time for everybody. You were such a remarkable support to Paul during the last two years. I hope that over the months to come you will take comfort in the knowledge that Paul was one of the finest ambassadors British sport has ever had. He was the most generous sportsman I have ever met. I hope that when my own son grows up, he will grow to play sport like Paul – fair but always in good spirit. I will never forget him Lindsey – he was a wonderful man.

With love to you and Evie
Graham Cowdrey
Public Relations Manager
Cantor Fitzgerald

Old friends of both mine and Paul's got in touch. One snooker chum from Paul's teenage years wrote from Tanzania, where he was teaching.

Unbreakable

Dear Lindsey

I just wanted to write to you to tell you how deeply sorry I am about the terrible news about Paul. He was a courageous, generous and wonderful human being who would grace any stage he was on. I remember being a very nervous teenager and going to meet him for the very first time. He was a fantastic prospect at the time and as soon as I met him he made me feel so welcome. He was so down to earth and never had a bad word to say about anybody – a character trait that has served him so well over the years. From 14 to 18 we were really close friends and although we had lost touch in recent years, whenever I saw him we still carried on as if we had seen each other a few days ago. He was so much fun to be around and had a cracking sense of humour. His talent was second to none and he has given millions of people many great memories. He lived life to the full … I would love to have seen him as a dad. I have watched him fundraise and fight courageously to battle his illness and this is something truly remarkable. My parents sent me newspaper clippings out to Tanzania where I am teaching, just to keep me updated on his fundraising – the pride I felt seeing him do this was immense. This gave me the inspiration to do something for the street kids of Tanzania. I last saw Paul just over a year ago when we had a round of golf. He was clearly in a lot of pain, but his sense of humour, strength of character and joy for life shone through. I will miss him greatly, I will remember him fondly and feel privileged to have so many happy memories of him.

Yours faithfully
Chris
Tanzania

The letters from fans were sometimes almost unbearable. There were many from children, often with a pound or two from their pocket money for the Paul Hunter Foundation, which had been set up in his name to allow underprivileged children the chance of playing snooker:

Dear Mrs Hunter
I'm sorry that Paul died after his fight for cancer. I idolized him as a snooker player and by using his talent he made a whole lot of people happier. Paul made this world a better place.
   Patrick, age 10
   County Tyrone

I was often amazed that our lives had touched so many people. I had some incredible letters from fans who had serious troubles of their own.

Dear Lindsey and Evie Rose
I must write and tell you how much Paul will be missed on the snooker circuit. He was a brilliant player and a wonderful ambassador for the game, on and off the table. But most of all, I will remember Paul with great affection for being a true gentleman and a family man, who had a word for everybody, whether he won or lost, and that is a very special quality as not all players have this gift. I have cerebral palsy. When Paul was diagnosed with his illness, I was extremely touched by his positive attitude and courage, and it never crossed my mind that Paul wouldn't get better. I will never forget Paul. Whenever I hear Atomic Kitten's 'Whole Again' I will always remember you

saying how he twirled you around in his bedroom and asked you
to marry him. I'm sure I speak for all snooker fans when I ask,
when you're feeling better, would you please write a book about
your life with Paul, as it will be a little keepsake for all snooker
fans to treasure. I know exactly what it is like to lose the most
important person in your life, young. I lost my dad when I was
17 and I lost my boyfriend to MS. God bless, my thoughts and
prayers will be with you and Paul and the family always.

    Love and best wishes
    Claire
    Rhondda

A 13-year-old fan from Germany wrote:

Dear Lindsey
Paul Hunter was a wonderful person whose smile never faded;
not even in hard times. I always admired him for the way he
saw a positive side of everything. But I also admire you though.
You have been a marvellous wife and mother in every situation,
even though the last 18 months must have been very difficult for
you. I find it unbelievable how well you dealt with the situation
and think you deserve a BIG praise. Paul couldn't have wished
for a better wife. Losing Paul is a big loss for you and the rest of
the family, but also for snooker and his millions of fans. He was
a real character with a mixture of the best of everything in him.
No one's as good or nice as Paul. It was my biggest wish, my
biggest dream to meet him one day and it's really hard for me
and hurts to accept that I will never be able to fulfil this dream.
Still, I won't ever forget him, because he was one of the nicest

*people I have ever heard of. God bless, Paul. He's my best
sportsman ever and that will NEVER change! May he rest in
peace. You and the family have all my sympathies and are
always, always in my thoughts, just like Paul.*

Love Alex

Even on holiday, people stopped what they were doing to
write to me.

Dear Mrs Hunter

*I'm here in Malta on holiday and heard the devastating news of
Paul's death. I cannot say how sorry I am. I've followed his
progress from his turning professional through his early Welsh
Open win in 1998 and been quite delighted with the British
Open win in 2002. He seemed such a lovely young guy – and
very genuine. I like following snooker and was especially pleased
to see such an honest 'no frills' player. On one occasion he told
the referee that he'd done a double hit – the TV hadn't picked it
up, nor had the referee or opponent. That, for me, showed a
TRUE SPORTSMAN and I respected him so dearly for it. My
thoughts and prayers go out to you and little Evie Rose, that you
will find the strength to get through.*

Yours sincerely
B M Smith
Malta

Other people thought of sharing memories with me in the
days after Paul's death.

Dear Mrs Hunter

We just felt we had to write to you to express our deepest sympathy at the very sad loss of your husband, Paul. We had seen him play many times at the Crucible, Sheffield, and met him a few times, of which, every time he was such a gentleman and had time for his fans. It was clear to see that Paul had everything it took to become a World Snooker Champion – sadly, time and illness prevented this, but he will remain a champion with snooker fans in all our hearts as I'm sure he will for you and your lovely daughter, Evie Rose. I too never knew my dad, like little Evie, but I never missed out on anything and the one thing I am grateful for is that I had such a loving and close relationship with my lovely mum, as I'm sure you will have and treasure those times together as I did.

 God Bless
 Wendy and Alan
 Shrewsbury

Hundreds of people had stories to tell of Paul's kindness and genuine interest in fans.

To the Hunter family
Please accept my heartfelt condolences in what must be the most difficult of times. I, like many others, was stunned to hear the news this week and feel that snooker has lost one of the true greats of the sport. I have been a huge fan of Paul's for many years and first contacted him seven years ago. I was shocked and surprised that he wrote a lovely letter back with a signed photo, and later that year a Christmas card. Having met him a few

times though, it was obvious that it was in his nature to make sure that he had enough time for his fans. Many times I've been at snooker tournaments and some players have just stormed out of the venue. But Paul, even after losing a match, would always stop to chat to people, sign autographs, have pictures taken, and always remembered a familiar face! I'll never forget that he managed to get my friend and I some tickets to the afternoon session at the Crucible – there was a massive queue at the box office and it was probably sold out! Although I followed snooker for many years before Paul came on the circuit, I never went to see a live match until he was playing in the late nineties. Some of the best (and most nerve-racking) nights of my life were watching those three Masters finals!

Yours
Zoe
Surrey

And some of the most poignant letters came from people who knew first-hand about what cancer is like.

Dear Lindsey
I was deeply saddened to hear of Paul's death. The tributes through this week will be of some comfort in the harrowing time – Paul was dearly loved by so many – and will be a treasured read over years to come. The courage and dignity with which he battled will long be remembered. I write as someone who lost his wife (Liddy) to NET cancer and as a team member at the NET Patient Foundation. One of Paul's 'legacies' is the wonderful website which is being of such great help and support

to so many. You both worked so hard to raise such significant funds and the leap forward is beyond our wildest dreams. Thank you. *Paul's death is beyond comprehension. The hurt will ease and you will treasure the memories.*

> *Yours*
> *Peter Gwilliam*
> *Surrey*

I thank all of the above for giving me permission to reprint their letters here, and I'd like to thank each and every person who wrote to me. Your letters comforted me more than you will ever know.

Unbreakable

If you would like to make a donation to the Paul Hunter NET Patient Foundation, you can do so at the website:

www.netpatientfoundation.com

or telephone 0800 434 6476.

If you would like to make a donation or apply for a grant to The Paul Hunter Foundation, you can do so at the website:

www.paulhunterfoundation.org

or email paulhunterfoundation@ntlworld.com

Acknowledgements

To Mum and Dad for bringing me up to be the sort of person I am. For never judging me and for always being there; for letting me be who I am; and for giving me the values that have seen me through and which I will now pass on to Evie.

To Tracy for being the greatest big sister in the world – everyone should have one like her! And to Chris, Matthew and Eloise for being the best uncle and cousins Evie could wish for. I thank you from the bottom of my heart for being so kind and so lovely to both of us, and for keeping life simple and fun for my baby – she will never be without a family who adores her as long as she has you all in her world.

To Nicky for introducing me to Paul, and for being there through all the ups and downs; you were Paul's cousin, but you've been my friend throughout. I want to thank Nobby and Mia too for including me in your family – all through your own bad times you've thought of me.

To my closest friends – Helen, Vicky, Sally, Mandy, and

Karen. You've been there for it all, and I appreciate so much the nights out, the support and the laughs, and the way you let me just be Lindsey.

To Brandon and Charlotte for going way beyond the bounds of what you were expected to do, and for becoming such good friends to me and to Paul.

To Paul's parents, Alan and Kris, who brought Paul into the world and made him the amazing character he was. Thanks to you, and to his sister Leanne and her husband Adam for sharing memories with me – I hope you'll always be there for Evie.

To Linda, my ghostwriter, and editor Gill Paul. It was actually lovely to spend all that time talking about Paul – I only wish you could have met him.

To everyone at HarperCollins who brought this book about.

To Kirkwood Hospice for all they did for Paul in his final days, and for being there for people who are living this now and will do so in the future.

Finally, to all Paul's fans. The support and kindness we received from the moment he was diagnosed was incredible. The thousands of letters, cards and messages that were sent showed what amazing loyalty and love he generated. If there is anyone who didn't receive a reply, please accept my apologies – and also, at this time, my thanks.

Lindsey Hunter
May 2007